Healthy Skin, Beautiful Skin

The 30-Day Nutritional Way

Healthy Skin, Beautiful Skin

The 30-Day Nutritional Way

Tere Ingram & Mark Hunter

Walker and Company   New York

To my mother
for her love
and support
—Tere

First published in the United States of America in 1985 by the Walker Publishing Company, Inc.

Published simultaneously in Canada by John Wiley & Sons Canada, Limited, Rexdale, Ontario.

Library of Congress Cataloging-in-Publication Data

Ingram, Tere.
   Healthy skin, beautiful skin.

   Bibliography: p.
   Includes index.
   1. Skin—Care and hygiene. 2. Skin—Diseases—Diet therapy—Popular works. 3. Skin—Diseases—Nutritional aspects—Popular works. I. Hunter, Mark. II. Title.
RL87.I54 1985   616.5   85-17947
ISBN 0-8027-0844-7
ISBN 0-8027-7287-0 (pbk.)

Printed in the United States of America

10 9 8 7 6 5 4 3 2 1

Text design by Laurie McBarnette

Contents

Chapter 8

Chapter 9

Chapter 10

Acknowledgment

To the United States Department of Agriculture, without whose extraordinary contributions to the hard statistical facts of nutrition, to the development of sound livable-with guidelines for good health, and to the creation of recipes that make food that's good for you taste good, this book would not have been possible. And to that pioneering breed of nutritional scientists who—despite scepticism from, and often repudiation by, conventional medical science—have in the last decade brought about a revolution in our approach to health. This book is a record of just one of their many path-breaking achievements.

Caution

This book is based on my experiences and the studies of nutritional and medical literature made by Mark Hunter and myself. It is not intended, nor should it be regarded, as medical advice. Before changing your diet, or adding supplements to it, consult your doctor. Only a doctor is qualified to treat skin disorders, or any other diseases.

—*Tere Ingram*

Introduction
The Program That Succeeded When Everything Else Failed

I'm Tere Ingram. This is my mother's story. It could be yours. It's about a skin ailment that no doctor could cure. But we curbed it together, my mother and I. What I learned changed our lives. It could change yours.

My mother, about ten years ago, woke up one morning to find patches of redness and sores all over her body. A woman who had taken her health for granted for forty or so years, she was upset, but she was sure the condition would clear up in a few days. It didn't.

What's causing it? she asked herself. Something different in my diet? She eliminated all foods except those she'd been eating all her adult life. No change. A laundry detergent? A soap? She switched brands. No change. Synthetic fabrics? She closeted her polyesters and dressed in wool, cotton, and silk. No change.

Weeks went by. No change.

She had a dreadful feeling that the sores were there to stay, that they wouldn't go away. She was afraid. She made an appointment with a dermatologist. He confirmed her fears. No, he told her, they wouldn't go away. She had a disease called psoriasis, and it was incurable. Yes, she was likely to have it for the rest of her life. "What caused it?" she wanted to know. "Why me?"

"We don't know," he said. "Maybe it's hereditary."

"But there's never been anybody in my family with psoriasis," she said.

He shrugged.

"What can you do for me?" my mother wanted to know.

"It's a relatively mild case," he said, "and we'll experiment together with some drugs to treat the symptoms."

She left the dermatologist's office with a prescription for a skin salve, a follow-up appointment slip, and a heavy burden of disappointment and grief. But, she hoped, maybe the salve would work. Surely the government wouldn't permit a doctor to prescribe a salve that didn't work. It didn't.

But my mom had faith in the medical profession, and so did I.

Somewhere there had to be a doctor who would know what to do; someplace there had to be a drug that, even if it couldn't cure, could help. I remember going with her to another doctor, sitting with her in his office, holding her hand, and thinking: Doctors study the human body for years and years and know everything there is to know about it. Surely one of them will understand what's going wrong inside of her and be able to cure it. Maybe this one will be *the* one. He wasn't.

Nor were any of the others, and there were many. Over the next few years, my mother spent thousands of dollars on doctors, on prescription drugs and nonprescription drugs, but nothing helped. There were creams to put on her sores, pills to swallow. Nothing helped. Some doctors told her to bathe with coal-tar soaps. They didn't tell her that coal tar could cause cancer. The soaps didn't help. No words of mine can describe the anguish and despair of a skin disease, the feeling that you've been marked as somebody different, inferior, for everybody to see. Simply going out to shop, to take a walk, to visit family and friends is an agony of self-consciousness, anxiety, and embarrassment. But nothing helped.

There was a long stretch then when she gave up on the medical profession, accepted her condition, and without complaint tried to lead a normal life. There were times during this period that her condition seemed to get better, and her hopes soared. She had heard about remissions of even cancer. Surely psoriasis could go away by itself, too. But it didn't. Perhaps, because of her frustration, perhaps because her faith in the medical profession had never died, she decided to see another doctor.

A friend of my mother's recommended a "good doctor." He was quite a distance away, and my mother hates to drive even short distances, but she went. Her first visit began, she told me, like all the first visits she had previously endured. Yes, she had psoriasis. No, there was no cure. But then this doctor said something none of the other doctors had said, and new hope flooded into my mother's heart. He said: With regular visits and treatment, he could keep her skin clear. Keep her skin clear! She could look well again, normal, go out without shame, enjoy being with people and not feel like running away and hiding.

She kept several appointments, eagerly. He prescribed cortisone creams and some over-the-counter coal-tar derivatives. Her sores seemed to get better, but not much. They did not clear up. Injections of cortisone followed. They changed my mother's personality. She became irritable, anxious, and eventually depressed. Things quickly went from bad to worse. The sores on her skin began to spread, open up, and bleed. She lost her appetite, took to her bed and stayed there because of extreme fatigue and deepening depression. When, in time, the effects of the cortisone wore off, she called the dermatologist and said, "Never again."

But more harm had been done by her years of treatments. She was finished with skin doctors, but not with other doctors. Her annual checkup revealed kidney damage and high blood pressure. Drainage of excess fluid in her kidneys, and a low-salt died supplemented with blood-pressure pills, corrected the condition. But that wasn't the end of the price her body was forced to pay for her years of psoriasis treatments.

One afternoon my sister Pat, a registered nurse, was swimming with Mom. Pat noticed a red spot on Mom's shoulder. Pat looked more closely at the spot and told her that it looked different from anything she had seen on her skin before. She said, "Mom, it just doesn't look like psoriasis to me." After years of working in hospitals, Pat had seen almost every kind of illness and had a great deal of experience with cancer. Not wanting to frighten Mom, she told her it probably wasn't cancer, but would she have it looked at just to be sure? But what if it was cancer? When my mother told me what Pat had said, I insisted she see a cancer specialist (an oncologist) at once.

My mother was lucky. Her oncologist turned out to be a good, kind man, and a superior doctor. What impressed my mother most about him was his interest in *her*. Not her symptoms, not her disease. *Her*. He spent a lot of time with her, asked penetrating questions about her past medical history, medications, feelings, family, and general lifestyle. From her answers, he seemed to think there was a chance of cancer, but he said honestly, "Mrs. Ingram, this spot on your shoulder looks very much like the psoriasis on your arm to me, but let's not do anything until we're sure. I'll take a tissue sample, send it to the lab and we'll see. This way, I'll feel better and so will you."

The lab said it was cancer.

It had probably developed during her psoriasis treatments. Her doctor told her it was basal cell cancer, and it could be cured by surgery. It was. But still, there was no cure for the psoriasis; and, to my mother's mind and mine, there might be danger from any further medical treatment for it.

That's when I decided to find the answers myself. I was trained as a nurse, and I know how to read scientific literature. That was the key, because every experiment, positive or negative, every bit of research conducted in clinics or laboratories that's worthy of being published, appears in scientific publications worldwide. If you know what you're looking for in that mass of print matter, you can find it. I did.

What I found was that there was a new, exciting branch of medicine growing up that said, in essence: Drugs are alien invaders of the body; they don't always cure, but they may always harm—there's another way: a nutritional way. I was amazed to discover that just switching over to the right selections from Food Groups designated by the United States Department of Agriculture, and supplementing them with vitamins and minerals, could turn unattractive skin into beautiful skin—and even prevent and curb skin diseases. Including psoriasis? Yes.

I put everything I dug out of the scientific literature into a palatable eating program for my mother. "You tried everything else," I told her, "Try this." She did.

If the definition of a fairy tale is a tragedy with a happy ending, then my mother's story is a fairy tale. Within a month on her new nutritious diet, she saw a definite improvement. Within six months, her sores had shrunk to pink patches. In a year's time, her skin was clear. What should not go unsaid is: That throughout my mother's long illness, I continually prayed to God to heal my mother's skin, and in His own time and in His own way, He answered my prayers.

After my mother's wonderful recovery, I felt I must learn more about the nutritional approach to good health and to good skin. I enlisted the support of Mark Hunter, a good friend, who dangles a Phi Beta Kappa key, worked for his doctorate in biochemistry, and is as skilled a medical-library researcher as you can find. I had another reason for joining up with Mark. I wanted to bring the good news about eating for beautiful skin to everybody, and Mark is one of the nation's top science ghost writers. In the last couple of years, he's researched and written three national diet and fitness best-sellers for celebrities' signatures—and that's only three of the fifty-five or so books he's had published.

Together, Mark and I culled, analyzed, appraised every scientific report on nutrition and the skin that we could feast our eyes on. And from those reports that seemed irrefutable, unassailable, duplicatable, and irreproachable, we designed a program—a simple, tasty one—to help you to beautiful skin, and to help prevent and curb skin diseases, and the damage done to your skin by stress, smoking, the Pill, sea and surf. Not the least fairy-tale-ish part of the program is that you can transform unattractive skin into beautiful skin in just 30 days. But no magic is involved; just sound nutrition. Here is, in brief outline:

The Eat for Beautiful Skin Program

It's the first and only skin-care program based on nutrition—without drugs, surgery, disagreeable therapies, or cover-up cosmetics.

One reason for its appeal is its 1-2-3 simplicity:

1. Start on the Eat for Beautiful Skin Menus and supplements today. (Chapter 3.)

2. Stay on the menus and supplements for the 30 days it takes for your body to replace unattractive skin with beautiful skin. (Learn about that in Chapter 1.)

3. Then apply The Nutritional Formula for Lifetime Beautiful Skin daily. (Chapter 4.)

By modifying your Eat for Beautiful Skin Menus and supplements you can help prevent and curb such skin diseases as acne, psoriasis, eczema, herpes, and premature aging; and the damages done to your skin by its enemies on the outside of your body and on the inside.

All the Eat for Beautiful Skin Program requires you to do is enjoy good-tasting, wholesome food that you can pluck from any supermarket shelf, augmented daily with nutrient supplements. The Eat for Beautiful Skin Recipes (Chapter 13) tell you how to make that good-tasting food taste even better.

It is important for you to know that this complete nutritional skin-care program, although derived from the verified, unassailable findings of authoritative nutritional scientists, has never been presented in its entirety before, and therefore must be regarded as experimental. It is published here for educational purposes, so you will be better equipped as an informed consumer to work with your doctor for the health and beauty of your skin.

I
Beautiful Skin in 30 Days

1 Beautiful Skin in 30 Days: The Nutritional Breakthroughs That Did It

Healthy skin glows.

It's dewy fresh. It's vibrant. It's the color of youth. It's vivacious. It's soft. It's fragrant. It's expressive, mirroring on your face your happiness and disapprovals, then relaxing into unruffled serenity. It's smooth. It's alive to the touch, warm, responsive.

It's attractive in the loveliest sense of the word: it pulls people to you, admiringly. It's sexy. It's satiny, shimmery, sleek. It's luminescent. It's sparkling. It ignores the years. It makes statements: positive ones, about your self-esteem, your sensuality. It has esprit.

Healthy skin is beautiful skin.

It can be yours. In 30 days.

Three breakthroughs in nutritional research in recent years have made it possible.

They concern not only the skin you see, but the layers hidden beneath it. It's in those layers that the skin's beauty is created. Beauty *is* skin-deep.

The hidden skin

On the next page is a diagram of a cross-section of the skin. Anatomically (how it's built) and functionally (what it does), the skin has been thoroughly explored by conventional medical science. (But how it works basically, as you shall see in this chapter and throughout the book, is the exclusive province of the nutritional scientist.) **1** on the diagram is the bottom layer of the epidermis, the basal cell layer. That's where the skin-cell "factory" is located. The skin cells produced in it rise through successive layers of the epidermis, growing, maturing, reaching their peak of health and beauty, and then dying at the uppermost region of the skin, **2**, the stratum corneum.

The dead skin cells are said to be keratinized. Keratin is the

THE HIDDEN SKIN

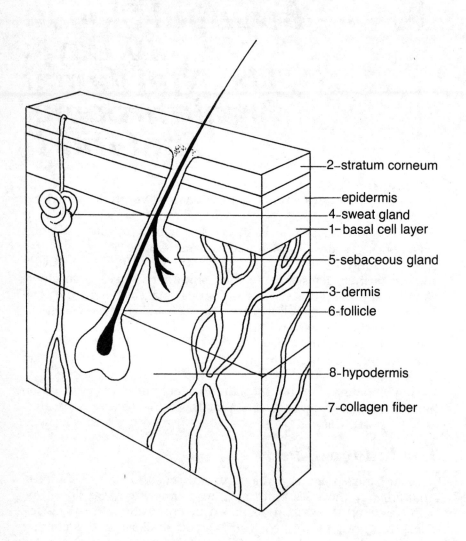

2–stratum corneum

epidermis

4–sweat gland

1– basal cell layer

5-sebaceous gland

3–dermis

6-follicle

8–hypodermis

7–collagen fiber

principal component of nails, horn, hair and the quills of feathers; and that gives you a good idea of what dead skin cells would look like *if* you could see them. Fortunately, they're normally microscopic and invisible. What you see are the new skin cells, pushing up beneath them and constantly rejuvenating the skin. But if your skin has that dull flaky look, the keratinized cells have accumulated in such numbers that you—and people looking at you—can see them as a mass; and it's time for soap and water, gentle scrubbing, and—most important, as you shall see—a change of diet.

Raw material for the skin-cell factory comes from the dermis, **3**, which contains a delivery network (blood vessels) a communications network (nerves and nerve endings), and a security network (lymph vessels). These don't appear in the diagram, because there are so many they would make the densest road map look like a model of clarity by comparison. The dermis also houses "factories" that in good health keep the skin cells in peak condition: sweat glands, **4**, which keep the skin cool by secreting water, and clean by eliminating wastes; sebaceous glands, **5**, which keep the skin supple by emitting a colorless, odorless, oily substance called sebum; and follicles **6**, which help keep the skin from minor dirt/dust/insect irritations with a protective coating of hair.

Protection from the harsh alkaline chemicals that are normal to most atmospheres (even in the millennia before modern industry) comes from an acid mantle formed by a compounding of the secretions of the oil and sweat glands. But for the mantle to work, the acidity must be just right: a pH of 5.5. pH is an indicator of acidity. A pH of 7 means neutral; above 7 means alkaline, the opposite of acid; below 7 means acid, and the lower the number the greater the acidity. When the skin is too acid, below a pH of 5.5, it begins to self-destruct. When it's not acid enough, above a pH of 5.5, it fails to protect against the alkaline chemicals in the atmosphere. Alkaline soaps can lift the skin's pH above 5.5, which is a good reason for staying away from them.

Collagen—that beautifying wonder of the cosmetic surgeon—is a natural substance in which the dermis abounds. It's made up of protein fibers—that's one of them at **7**—that you can think of as extraordinarily elastic, resilient rubber strips. They hold the skin together, yet permit it to move as the body moves and bounce back into place as the body rests, unfatigued, fresh, unmarked.

That's what cosmeticians call tone. Your skin has it when your collagen hasn't stiffened like an old rubber hose—and your skin, in consequence, hasn't sagged and wrinkled, and stiffened, too—under the assaults of collagen's many enemies, not the least of which is the sun. To protect collagen against the sun's pernicious ultraviolet rays, at the base of the epidermis is the body's own sunscreen—the dark skin pigment, melanin. But in point of fact, it doesn't do a very good job; and diet and manmade sunscreens have to come to the rescue (that's in Chapter 12).

Cushioning the dermis—at **8**—is the hypodermis (the word means under the dermis), a fatty tissue that supports, rounds out, and contours the skin. Take away a good deal of its fat rapidly, as many of us do when we crash-diet, and that support, and the rounding-out and contouring crashes, too, leaving a sagging, formless sac of a skin. Fat overall isn't beautiful, but without fat your skin can't be beautiful. That's just one reason the successful approach to skin beauty is through nutrition.

The other reasons become clear when you examine the three nutritional breakthroughs that can lead to beautiful skin.

Breakthrough 1:
The skin is a nutritional system

Don't regard the skin as an organ (it is, the biggest in the body). Don't regard the skin as a breathing machine (it is, taking in its own oxygen and spewing out its own carbon dioxide). Don't regard the skin as your firstline of defense against the hostile world out there (it is for all its beauty an obdurate shield for the soft, fragile organs, tissues and vessels within). Don't regard the skin as a thermostat (it is, holding your body temperature within the norms of healthy life). Don't regard your skin as an antidote for poisons (it is, ridding your body of some wastes that would otherwise kill it).

Regard your skin the new way: as a system.

A baseball team is an example of a system. It's composed of nine men. Each has a specific job. The first baseman covers first base; the second baseman, second; the third baseman, third. The outfielders divide responsibility for right, center and left field. The pitcher pitches; the catcher catches. The shortstop patrols the grass between second and third. Each player takes his turn at bat. A baseball team wins when all members play together, and it's strong in every position. One superstar won't make a winner, two superstars won't make a winner, when all or most of the other members of the team are weak. Every player must contribute winning baseball.

The skin is a system composed of nutrients. Each has a specific job to do. But it can't do it without the aid of the other nutrients, just as a baseball player is useless without the other members of his team. Vitamin A is a skin-system superstar; but add it to your diet, say, to help prevent acne, and do nothing about strengthening the other nutrients in the system, and you won't curb acne. Investigators who checked the behavior of another nutritional superstar in another of the body's systems, made a similar discovery: Yes, you can prevent the common cold with vitamin C when all other nutrients in the immune system are at top strength. And, no, you can't when they're not.

The practical guideline arising from the systems approach to the skin is this: To create winning skin—healthy and beautiful—consume the right foods and supplements to give the skin system the nutrients it needs at top strength. What those nutrients are, and how we know we're getting them at top strength, was discovered through another nutritional breakthrough.

Breakthrough 2:
The skin's nutrient team

When nutritional scientists deprived the skin of vitamin A, they found it wouldn't grow properly and it bungled its repairs. When they held back on vitamin B_5, they discovered the skin grew lazy about manufacturing the fats and oils it needs. When they decreased the daily quota of manganese, they learned that the skin had trouble breathing. When they rationed the supply of linoleic acid, they noted that the skin went dry. By numerous deprivation experiments such as these, nutritional scientists have identified the nutrients the skin system can't do without—the members of the skin's nutrient team. The complete roster appears on the following page. *Although it contains forty-two nutrients, you can obtain all of them with a sensible and delicious diet supplemented with just one multivitamin-mineral product* (see page 14).

Nutritional scientists then made an unexpected discovery. The roster of the skin's nutrient team and the rosters of the nutrient teams of all the other systems in the body—cardiovascular, im-

THE SKIN'S NUTRIENT TEAM

Vitamin A
Vitamins of the B
  Complex
  Vitamin B_1
  Vitamin B_2
  Vitamin B_3
  Vitamin B_5
  Vitamin B_6
  Vitamin B_{12}
  Folic acid
  Biotin
  Inositol
  Choline
  PABA

Vitamin C with Bioflavinoid
  Complex
Vitamin D
Vitamin E
Minerals
  Calcium
  Chromium
  Copper
  Iodine
  Iron
  Magnesium

Manganese
Molybdenum
Phosphorus
Potassium
Selenium
Zinc

Essential fatty acids
  Linoleic acid
  Linolenic acid
  Arachidonic acid

Essential amino acids
  Isoleucine
  Leucine
  Lysine
  Methionine
  Phenylalanine
  Threonine
  Tryptophan
  Valine

Nucleic acids
Fats
Carbohydrates
Proteins

mune, nervous, visual, reproductive and so on—are identical. They differ only in the top strengths required of corresponding nutrients. For example, the skin system requires a higher top strength for vitamin A than the cardiovascular system, and the nervous system requires a higher top strength for vitamins of the B complex than the reproductive system.

"Top strength" means the optimal—the right—amount of a nutrient in a system. What those optimal amounts are for the nutrients in each system of the body, including the skin's, are not yet known. But what is known are the optimal amounts required to keep the whole body at the peak of wellness. When the body receives those amounts, a regulatory mechanism at the base of the brain (the *hypothalamus*) distributes optimal shares to each of the body's systems. So by consuming optimal amounts of nutrients for the whole body, you automatically consume optimal amounts for each of the body's systems, including the skin's system.

The optimal amounts of nutrients required by the body are called the RDA's, the Recommended Daily Allowances. (You'll find the numbers in the chart on page 15.) They're the basis for the health of your body, and the health and beauty of your skin. Consume less than your RDA's, and, although you may not exhibit symptoms of a disease, you're not as well as you could be—and neither is your skin.

Breakthrough 3:
Unattractive skin is a nutrient-deficiency disease

Unattractive skin is dull, drab, rough, lacking in resiliency, dry or oily (and sometimes both at the same time, in different parts of the skin), tired-looking, lackluster, blah. Go to a doctor with it, and he'll tell you there's nothing wrong; and, based on his training, he'll have made the right diagnosis: unattractive skin shows no clinical symptoms of any known illness. And yet you're ill. Unattractive skin is a member of a newly discovered group of symptomless diseases.

That's a new idea, and it needs to be explained in a new way, with this variation of the Ainsworth continuum (named after its inventor, Dr. Thomas H. Ainsworth, a former director of the American Hospital Association):

H_____D

H is the highest level of wellness. D is the lowest: terminal illness and death.

H_____D
                        O

O is the onset of illness, which in the case of skin disorders is manifested at first microscopically. It is not until the appearance of blatant symptoms, S,

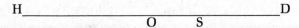

ranging from whiteheads to psoriasis and cancer lesions, that the dermatologist draws on his/her armamentarium of abrasives, drying soaps, disinfectants, peeling medicines and drugs to bring the patient back to a state

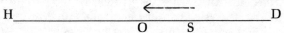

just a bit before the onset of the illness. But that's a long way from the highest level of wellness. Preceding the onset of disease, there's a stretch of time, indicated by slanting lines on the continuum, during which there are no clinical symptoms, but

H_____ /////////////// _____D
          O   S

during which you are no longer healthy. It's the period of symptomless diseases. It's during this period that your skin is unattractive.

Symptomless diseases (some are: mood swings, fatigue, weight gain, weakness, irritability, poor reflexes, memory lapses, digestive upsets, anxiety and just plain feeling rotten—all lowlevel) have been associated with nutrient deficiencies. Unattractive skin, a symptomless disease, is a nutrient-deficiency disease.

Nutrient deficiency means you're not consuming your RDA's. That's not hard to do. Junk food is nutrient-impoverished. Most foods are grown with chemical antagonists of nutrients; are plucked before they can ripen into their full quota of nutrients; and are decimated of nutrients by shipping, storage, packaging, freezing, processing and chemical additives. We eat empty calories, like white sugar, that contribute zero nutrients. We eat dangerous calories, like saturated fats, that convert in the body into havoc-creating chemicals (oxidants and others) that savage nutrients. We expose ourselves to conditions and substances that deplete the nutrient store in our bodies—stress, smoking, the Pill, sun and surf, pollutants in air, water and food. We, ironically, take some medicines to make us well that annihilate nutrients.

Little wonder, then, that the U.S. Department of Agriculture admits that on the average American diet most American women can't get even their RDA's of some nutrients. But you *can* get your RDA's. And when you do, you're on your way to . . .

Beautiful skin in 30 days

You can get your RDA's with a proper diet—free of empty calories, dangerous calories, and other nutrient busters—properly supplemented. Supplementation is necessary because the products of today's agribusiness are so deficient in nutrient values that even on a scrupulously balanced diet of wholesome foods, you can't get some of your RDA's.

With a sound, supplemented diet—the kind of diet your Eat for Beautiful Skin Menus provide (see Chapters 3 and 4)—you can restore unattractive skin to the highest level of wellness—

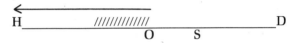

glowing, brightly hued, smooth, resilient, not oily, but moist and fresh. And you can do it in 30 days.

That's not because nutrients are wonder drugs (they're not drugs of any kind; they're foods) but because the right nutrients in the right amounts create healthy, beautiful skin cells; and it takes 30 days from the start of production at the base of the epidermis for them to rise to the surface of the skin. Mega-millions of them then push out the old cells and mesh together to form a new skin—the kind of skin you've always wanted.

2

The 52 Best Foods for Beautiful Skin— and the 52 Worst

Eating isn't only a matter of nutrients. If it were, you could pop vitamin and mineral pills, and never sit down to a meal again. To food lovers, what an abominable thought! Fortunately, eating is also a matter of energy. We love, work, play, create, run marathons, and run the gamut of emotions powered by the energy in our food. We must eat. And for beautiful skin, we must eat right.

Eating right means, to begin with, eating food that supplies energy. You can't subsist on no-cal drinks, because a cal(orie) is a measure of energy, and no-cal means no energy. You also can't subsist on them because their nutrient density—the variety and quantity of nutrients per calorie—is also 0. If you can't subsist on them, neither can your skin. That's why no-cal drinks are on the list of The 52 worst foods for beautiful skin.

What's on the list of The 52 best foods for beautiful skin are just the opposite of no-cal drinks. They have calories, but just enough to run your body system beautifully and keep your skin beautiful without adding an ounce to your weight. Their nutrient densities are about as high as you can get. To arrive at these 52 bests, we tracked down the 20 best food sources of each of the 42 nutrients mandatory for beautiful skin; and then from those hundreds of elite edibles, we selected the 52 with the highest nutrient densities.

Take the top 10 of the best 52, and you'll find that salmon is rich in 11 of the 42 nutrients the skin needs; eggs, in 13; rice, in 12; peas, in 10; walnuts, in 13; alfalfa, in 10; lentils, in 12; peanuts, in 10; sunflower seeds, in 13; and liver in 15—besides being adequately stocked with most of the rest. Sardines, a splendid food for the skin because it's the richest source of much-needed nucleic acids, is a runner-up to the top ten with an 8. These ingredients are good eating, tasty and (with the exception of alfalfa) familiar; and they're right for you and your skin.

The 52 worst are, as you can expect, wrong for you and your skin. Except for no-cal drinks, they all have calories, but most have

The 52 best foods for beautiful skin

Fruit
  Citrus fruits
  (orange, grapefruit, lemon,
    lime)
  Papaya
  Pineapple
  Strawberries

Vegetables
  Alfalfa
  Asparagus
  Avocado
  Cabbage
  Lentils
  Mushrooms
  Parsley
  Peas
  Spinach
  Sprouts
  Tomatoes

Whole grains
(including low- and no-sugar
  cereals and baked goods
  made with them)
  Barley
  Corn
  Oats
  Rice
  Rye
  Wheat
  Wheat germ

Milk/Cheese
  All cheeses
  (low-fat preferred)
  Skim milk
  Low-fat, low- or no-sugar
    yogurt

Beans
  All beans (especially chick-
  peas, pinto beans and
  soybeans)

Eggs
  (limit: three a week)

Fish and Seafood
  Flounder
  Halibut
  Herring
  Oysters
  Salmon
  Sardines
  Shrimp
  Tuna

Meat/Poultry
  Beef
  Chicken
  Lamb
  Liver
  Pork
  Veal

Oils
  Olive oil
  Sesame oil
  Sunflower oil

Nuts
  Almonds
  Brazil nuts
  Hazelnuts
  Peanuts
  Pecans
  Walnuts

Seeds
  Pumpkin seeds
  Sesame seeds
  Sunflower seeds

The 52 worst foods for beautiful skin*

Bologna
Cakes
Candies
Canned fruit
Capon
Chocolate
Chocolate drinks
Cocoa
Coconuts
Coconut oil
Coffee
Cookies
Corned beef
Custard
Deep-fried foods
Duck
Frankfurters
Frozen meals
Goose
Hydrogenated fats
Ice cream
Ice milk
Ices
Jams
Jellies
Ketchup
Lard
Liverwurst and other
  wursts
Margarine
Meats, fatty
Milk drinks
Nuts, roasted in oil and
  salted
No-Cal drinks
Palm oil
Pastrami

Pastries
Pies
Popcorn, salted
Potato chips
Preserves
Puddings
Salami
Sausages
Sherbets
Soft drinks, sugar-
  sweetened
Soups, canned
Sour cream
Smoked foods
Sweet cream
Tea
Thick shakes
Tongue

*Commercial nondietetic foods

too many per ounce for girth control; and most of the calories are empty and dangerous, adding nothing to your nutrient pool and deciminating the nutrients in it. Tastewise, the 52 worst are delightful; but skinwise, they're a disaster.

The 52 worst are arranged here alphabetically for easy reference. It's a good idea to keep the list handy (a reduced-size Xerox could help) when you shop for food or eat out; and when you review, as you should right now, the contents of your fridge and kitchen shelves. A larder devoid of the 52 worst is one of the first steps toward beautiful skin.

The second is a larder filled to the brim with the best 52. They're listed here alphabetically under food groups—fruit, whole grains, fish, beans and so on—because by making selections from those groups according to a formula developed by the U.S. Department of Agriculture, you can create the Eat for Beautiful Skin Menus, which are the final step toward beautiful skin. We've created those Menus for you in the next chapter; and we'll show you how you can do it yourself in the chapter after that.

But for starters, get used to the idea that there *are* foods that are good for your skin, and that they *should* replace foods that are bad for your skin. It's a mindset to ease you hassle-free into making the diet change that can give you beautiful skin.

3

The 30-Day Eating Plan with the Eat for Beautiful Skin Menus

Stay on these menus as they are, or modified to your taste, for 30 days, then look in the mirror, or in other people's eyes, and you'll want to stay on them for the rest of your lives. Both of us have stayed with them and can testify how wonderful our skin feels and looks.

The menus—three meals a day, snacking permitted, for seven days—are an orchestration of selections from The 52 Best Foods for Beautiful Skin, a few other good-for-your-skin foods, and one or two permissibles. They were composed in accordance with the United States Department of Agriculture's Daily Food Guide—a formula for obtaining a nutritious diet by making the right number of choices from the right food groups. (You'll learn how to apply this formula yourself in the next chapter.)

But as nutritious as the menus are—properly proportioned for fats, carbohydrates and proteins, and dense with other nutrients—they're the victims of modern agribusiness's nutrient-busting ways. Some of the menu ingredients are so below their nutrient norms that the menus on the whole can't provide you with some of your RDA's of some nutrients—the amounts your body needs for its health, and your skin needs for its health and beauty. Supplements are necessary.

You can get complete supplementation in almost any multivitamin-mineral ("one-a-day") product. The nutrient values set by the chart of Your Basic Supplement Needs for Beautiful Skin on the following page fulfill the RDA needs of most people on the Eat for Beautiful Skin Menus.

Check supplement labels against that chart to be certain you're getting all the necessary nutrients in the right range of values. If any nutrients are missing, purchase them separately. Do not exceed maximum values set by the chart. Vitamins and minerals are effective in extremely small quantities; and more is not always better. Excessive quantities of some vitamins and minerals may be dangerous.

A word about nutrient numbers: The amounts of nutrients that

YOUR BASIC FOOD SUPPLEMENT NEEDS FOR BEAUTIFUL SKIN

A single multivitamin-mineral product may help provide RDA's for most people on the Eat for Beautiful Skin Menus. To determine your individual supplement needs, consult your doctor.

Vitamin A   10,000 IU's
Vitamins of the B complex
  Vitamin B_1 2 mg.
  Vitamin B_2 2 mg.
  Vitamin B_3 20 mg.
  Vitamin B_5 10 mg.
  Vitamin B_6 2 mg.
  Vitamin B_{12} 4 mcg.
  Folic acid   2 mg.
  Biotin   5 mg.
  Inositol   100 mg.
  Choline   300 mg.
  PABA   50 mg.

Vitamin C with
  Bioflavinoids   500 mg.
Vitamin D   400 IU's
Vitamin E   100 IU's

Minerals
  Calcium   1,200 mg.
  Chromium   100 mcg.
  Copper   2 mg.
  Iodine   150 mcg.
  Iron   20 mg.
  Magnesium   1,000 mg.
  Manganese   10 mg.
  Molybdenum   100 mcg.
  Phosphorus   1,500 mg.
  Potassium   3,500 mg.
  Selenium   50 mcg.
  Zinc   15 mg.

Essential fatty acids
  Linoleic acid   *
  Linolenic acid   *
  Arachidonic acid   *

Essential amino acids
  Isoleucine   *
  Leucine   *
  Lysine   *
  Methionine   *
  Phenylalanine   *
  Threonine   *
  Tryptophan   *
  Valine   *

Nucleic acids   *
Fats   *
Carbohydrates   *
Proteins   *

* Optimal quantities supplied by the Eat-for-Beautiful-Skin Menus.

There are 454 grams in an ounce; a milligram (mg.) is a thousandth part of a gram; a microgram (mcg.), a millionth. An IU (International Unit) is a measure of the biological activity of a vitamin.

are right for *you* are right *only* for you; but what is right only for you is difficult if not impossible to determine at the present stage of nutritional knowledge. It's up to you, under the supervision of your doctor, to settle on the quantities that make you feel better and look better.

Here's how to use the Eat for Beautiful Skin Menus:

1. Start tomorrow morning.

2. Do not add anything to the menus, with one exception: There's no limit on added herbs and spices. Stay away, in particular, from foods on the list of The 52 Worst Foods for Beautiful Skin, or any foods resembling them.

3. For the first seven days, try to stay on the menus as they are to get the feel of them. But if you find any food objectionable, substitute an equivalent from the list of The 52 Best Foods for Beautiful Skin.

4. During the next twenty-three days, you can swap daily menus: Day 1 for Day 3, for example; or swap daily meals: Day 1 Breakfast for Day 3 Breakfast, for example. This helps dispel the boredom of oh-it's-Tuesday-and-it's-tuna-fish-again—a deadly enemy to anybody trying to stay on a new diet.

5. After the first thirty days, make up your own menus, with about a hundred more good-for-the-skin foods that you'll find listed in the next chapter. Instructions are there as well for creating your own menus.

A final word to weight-worriers: The Eat for Beautiful Skin Menus contribute between 1,200 and 1,500 calories. That's a maintenance diet for most women, and a reducing diet for some. If, after the first week, your scale shows a weight gain or loss, adjust the menus by decreasing or increasing portion sizes.

EAT FOR BEAUTIFUL SKIN MENUS

DAY 1

BREAKFAST

½ cup	fresh pineapple chunks
¾ cup	hot oatmeal with cinnamon, sprinkled with:
1 tablespoon	wheat germ
1 cup	skim milk
1 slice	whole-wheat toast with:
½ teaspoon	butter
1 teaspoon	honey

LUNCH

1	chicken sandwich, consisting of:
2 to 3 ounces	cooked chicken
2 slices	rye or whole-wheat bread
1 portion	coleslaw
1	orange

DINNER

2 to 3 ounces	broiled halibut with minced garlic, garnished with parsley
½ cup	steamed peas sprinkled with fresh herbs
¾ cup	brown rice, preferably cooked in chicken broth
1 cup	yogurt, with fruit

SNACK
Sunflower seeds, unsalted

DAY 2

BREAKFAST

½	fresh papaya or 1 orange
2	poached eggs
1 slice	whole-wheat toast
1 teaspoon	honey
1 cup	skim milk

LUNCH

1	tuna-fish sandwich consisting of:
1½ ounces	canned tuna fish
2 slices	rye or whole-wheat bread
1 large bowl	salad consisting of assorted salad greens, tossed with:
2 tablespoons	vegetable-oil dressing
½	grapefruit sweetened with honey if desired

DINNER

1½ ounces	sautéed calves' liver with onions
¾ cup	spaghetti with pepper and minced fresh herbs of your choice
½ cup	steamed fresh spinach with minced garlic
2-inch cube	cheddar or any savory cheese

SNACK

Sesame seeds

DAY 3

BREAKFAST

½ cup	strawberries with:
1 cup	cottage cheese, dry curd, low-fat, sprinkled with
1 tablespoon	wheat germ
1 slice	whole-wheat bread

LUNCH

2 to 3 ounces	canned or fresh salmon with lemon juice
1 large bowl	salad greens including spinach and sprouts, with:
2 tablespoons	vegetable or olive oil dressing
2 slices	rye or whole wheat bread
1 cup	yogurt with fruit

DINNER

2 to 3 ounces	broiled baby lamb chop with chives or tarragon, garnished with parsley
½ cup	fresh peas
½ cup	mushrooms
¾ cup	brown rice sprinkled with nutmeg
½ ounce	dessert cheese of your choice

SNACK

Almonds

DAY 4

BREAKFAST

½ cup	fresh papaya chunks or ½ grapefruit
¾ cup	hot cream of wheat with cinnamon, topped with:
½ cup	plain yogurt sprinkled with:
1 tablespoon	wheat germ

LUNCH

2 to 3 ounces	canned sardines, sprinkled with lemon juice, garnished with parsley
1 large bowl	salad consisting of alfalfa, sprouts and onions, tossed with:
2 tablespoons	vegetable or olive oil dressing
2 slices	rye or whole wheat bread
½ cup	mixed orange and grapefruit chunks

DINNER

1 cup	lentil soup
2 to 3 ounces	sautéed filet of flounder with garlic and herbs of your choice, sprinkled with lemon juice, and garnished with parsley
¾ cup	enriched white rice cooked in chicken stock
1 large bowl	chick-pea salad with sliced onions and mushrooms, tossed with:
1 tablespoon	vegetable oil dressing
3-inch cube	dessert cheese of your choice

SNACK

Unsalted peanuts

DAY 5

BREAKFAST

1	orange or ½ grapefruit
1	scrambled egg in nonstick skillet,
1	bagel (preferably whole-wheat), with:
1 cup	cottage cheese, dry-curd, low-fat

LUNCH

3 medium	cold boiled shrimp sprinkled with lime juice
1 large bowl	salad consisting of sprouts, alfalfa, mushrooms and onions, tossed with:
2 tablespoons	vegetable and olive oil dressing
1 slice	rye or whole-wheat bread
1 cup	skim milk

DINNER

2 to 3 ounces	broiled veal chop with garlic and herbs, garnished with parsley
½ cup	steamed spinach and minced onions
½ cup	corn kernels with pimentos
½ cup	fresh pineapple chunks, with:
½ cup	plain, low-fat yogurt

SNACK

Sunflower seeds

DAY 6

BREAKFAST

½ cup	fresh papaya chunks or ½ grape-fruit
1 ounce	puffed rice, with:
1 cup	skim milk, sprinkled with
1 tablespoon	wheat germ
1 slice	whole-wheat bread with:
1 teaspoon	honey

LUNCH

3	oysters on the half shell, sprinkled with lemon or lime juice
1 large bowl	salad consisting of spinach, mushrooms and onions, with:
1 tablespoon	vegetable oil dressing
1 slice	rye or whole-wheat bread

DINNER

1 cup	beef broth
¾ cup	soybeans
¾ cup	brown rice
¼ cup	sautéed mushrooms in nonstick skillet, with:
½ cup	steamed cabbage with garlic and herbs of your choice
¼ cup	fresh pineapple chunks, with:
2-inch cube	dessert cheese of your choice

SNACK

Walnuts

DAY 7

BREAKFAST

½ cup	mixed fresh pineapple, orange and papaya (optional) chunks
2 to 3 ounces	kippered herring
1	breakfast roll, whole-wheat or rye
2-inch cube	Swiss cheese

LUNCH

1 large bowl	health-food-store-type salad, consisting of sprouts, alfalfa, spinach, mushrooms and parsley, with:
1 tablespoon	vegetable and olive oil dressing
1 cup	skim milk

DINNER

1 cup	thick barley-mushroom soup
2 to 3 ounces	broiled pork chop with shallots and herbs of your choice, garnished with parsley
¾ cup	corn kernels cooked with onions
½ cup	spinach sautéed in nonstick skillet
½	baked grapefruit sweetened with:
1½ teaspoons	honey

SNACK
Sesame seeds

4 The Nutritional Formula for Lifetime Beautiful Skin

Here for the first time, the twenty best sources of each of the forty-two nutrients necessary for beautiful skin are arranged in six food groups: the Eat for Beautiful Skin Food Groups.* By making selections from each food group according to a basic formula developed by the U.S. Department of Agriculture nutritionists, you can create daily menus of favorite supermarket foods that provide maximum nutrition value not only for your skin but also for your whole body.

We used that formula to create the Eat for Beautiful Skin Menus from the best fifty-two foods in the six food groups. After you've been on the Eat for Beautiful Skin Menus for thirty days (or longer, if you choose), you can apply the same formula to the several hundred foods in the Eat for Beautiful Skin Food Groups to create your own Eat for Beautiful Skin Menus. They'll help keep your skin healthy and beautiful for the rest of your life.

This is the nutritional formula for lifetime beautiful skin:

• Four basic servings daily from the Fruit/Vegetable Food Group for Beautiful Skin (page 26). Count as a basic serving: ½ cup, or a typical portion, such as 1 orange, or ½ medium grapefruit or cantaloupe, juice of 1 lemon, a wedge of lettuce, a bowl of salad, and 1 medium potato.

• Four basic servings daily from the Whole Grains Food Group for Beautiful Skin (page 28). Count as a basic serving: 1 slice bread; ½ to ¾ cup cooked cereal, cornmeal, macaroni, spaghetti, noodles, or rice; or 1 ounce ready-to-eat cereal. Count a roll or bagel as 2 basic servings.

• Two basic servings daily from the Milk/Cheese Food Group for Beautiful Skin (page 28). Count as a basic serving: 1 cup (8 ounces) skim milk; 1 cup plain yogurt (low-fat); a 2-inch cube of hard

---

*For The 20 Best Sources of Selected Essential Nutrients for Beautiful Skin, see Appendix, page 145.

cheese; 2 ounces of soft cheese (including spreads); 4 tablespoons grated cheese; or 2 cups of cottage cheese.

• Two basic servings daily from the Meat/Poultry/Fish/Beans Food Group for Beautiful Skin, which also includes eggs, nuts, and seeds (page 27). Count as a basic serving: 2 to 3 ounces of lean cooked meat, poultry, fish, or seafood; 1 egg; ½ to ¾ cup cooked dry beans, dry peas, soybeans, or lentils; or ½ to 1 cup of nuts or seeds.

• As many servings as required daily for cooking and salad preparation from the oils of the Oils/Sweets Food Group for Beautiful Skin (page 28). Oils in this group are of vegetable origin only, since they contain more polyunsaturated than saturated fats. Saturated fats, often empty calories, are dangerous calories when eaten in excess, contributing to heart attack and other degenerative diseases, as well as unattractive skin. Polyunsaturated fats may become carcinogenic (cancer-producing) unless prevented by a team of protective nutrients. That protective team is present in the menu-supplement combinations suggested in this book. There are no specific basic servings for the sweets in this group, but use them sparingly as in the Eat for Beautiful Skin Menus.

• There is no limit on the servings in the Herbs/Spices Food Group for Beautiful Skin. Regarded until recently by conventional medical science as nonnutritive condiments, herbs and spices are now known, thanks mainly to comprehensive chemical analyses conducted by the U.S. Department of Agriculture, to be replete with essential vitamins and minerals. They also contribute substances that fight destructive biochemicals (oxidants and their derivatives) that attack all cells in the body, including the skin's.

Garlic is not only the most nutritionally potent food in this group (it's an herb), but, used judiciously, it also can be a culinary delight. There's widening acceptance by conventional doctors of this popular herb's preventive medical properties. A clove of garlic a day may help keep your dermatologist away.

Your Eat-for-Beautiful-Skin Menus (those we've created for you, and those you create for yourself from the nutritional formula for lifetime beautiful skin) conform to the Federal Dietary Guidelines for Americans developed jointly by the Departments of Health and Human Services and Agriculture. The Menus provide a variety of foods; help keep your weight down; are free of too much fats, saturated fats and cholesterol; contain optimal amounts of complex carbohydrates and fiber; and reduce the intake of salt and white sugar. They provide about 1,200 to 1,500 calories a day and can be adjusted to prevent excessive weight loss or gain by increasing or decreasing portion sizes. This type of diet not only fights bad skin but also, according to the United States Department of Agriculture, can help prevent heart attack, diabetes and other degenerative diseases. Your Eat for Beautiful Skin Menus may well be among the most nutritious and healthful available to adult Americans.

But, sadly, our agribusiness products by and large are nutrient-poor, can't supply most of the RDA's, and must be supplemented. Augment the Menus *you* create with the same multivitamin-mineral product (and additional products if necessary) with which you supplemented the Menus we created for you.

THE FRUIT/VEGETABLE FOOD GROUP FOR BEAUTIFUL SKIN

Fruits
Apricots
Bananas
Cantaloupe
Currants, black
Grapefruit
Guavas
Kumquats
Lemons
Limes
Oranges
Papayas
Persimmons
Strawberries

Vegetables
Alfalfa
Asparagus
Avocados
Beets
Broccoli
Cabbage
Carrots
Chard
Chives

Collard Greens
Dandelion greens
Eggplant
Endives
Green beans
Lentils
Mung beans
Mushrooms
Mustard greens
Onions, green
Parsley
Peas
Peppers, green
Peppers, red
Pimientos
Potatoes
Romaine lettuce
Spinach
Split peas
Sprouts, mature
Squash, winter
Tomatoes
Turnip greens
Watercress
Yams

THE MEAT/POULTRY/FISH/BEANS FOOD GROUP FOR BEAUTIFUL SKIN

(including eggs, nuts and seeds)

Meat
Beef
Kidneys
Lamb
Liver
Pork
Rabbit
Veal

Poultry
Chicken
Turkey

Fish/Seafood
Anchovies
Bass
Caviar
Clams
Cod
Crab
Eel
Flounder
Haddock
Hake
Halibut
Herring
Lobster
Mackerel
Mussels
Octopus
Oysters
Sablefish
Salmon
Sardines
Scallops
Scrod
Shark
Shrimp
Smelt
Snails
Snapper
Sole
Squid
Swordfish
Trout
Tuna
Whitefish

Beans
All beans, especially:
Pinto
Soybeans

Eggs
Soft-cooked preferred,
not to exceed three a week

Nuts
Almonds
Brazil nuts
Cashews
Hazelnuts
Peanuts
Pecans
Pistachios
Walnuts

Seeds
Sesame seeds
Pumpkin seeds
Sunflower seeds

THE WHOLE-GRAINS FOOD GROUP FOR BEAUTIFUL SKIN

(including low- and no-sugar cereals; pasta and baked goods made from whole grain)
Barley
Bran
Brewer's yeast
Buckwheat
Corn
Millet
Oats
Rice
Rice bran
Rice germ
Rye
Wheat
Wheat germ

THE MILK/CHEESE FOOD GROUP FOR BEAUTIFUL SKIN

Cheeses (low-fat preferred)
Milk, skim
Yogurt (low-fat, low- or no-sugar preferred)

THE OILS/SWEETS FOOD GROUP FOR BEAUTIFUL SKIN

Oils
Almond oil
Apricot oil
Cottonseed oil
Linseed oil
Olive oil
Safflower oil
Sesame oil

Soy oil
Sunflower oil
Walnut oil

Sweets
Blackstrap molasses
Carob
Honey

THE 12 BEST SOURCES OF POLYUNSATURATED FATS IN VEGETABLE OILS AND SALAD DRESSINGS

How to use this chart: The key figures are listed in the *Rating* column. The higher the rating, the higher the share of polyunsaturated fat in the product. The numbers in the other columns represent the milligrams of each type of fat in one tablespoon of the product.

| | FATS | | |
Vegetable oils	Polyun-saturated	Saturated	Rating
Corn	8.0	1.7	5
Cottonseed	7.1	3.5	2
Peanut	4.3	2.3	2
Soybean	7.9	2.0	4
Mixed (mostly soybean, with some cottonseed)	6.5	2.4	3
Sunflower	8.9	1.4	6
Olive	1.1	1.8	1
Salad Dressings			
Mayonnaise	5.7	1.6	4
Mayonnaise-type	2.6	.7	4
Italian	4.1	1.0	4
Blue cheese	4.3	1.5	3
French	3.4	1.5	2
Thousand Island	3.1	.9	3

Note: Although olive oil has the poorest rating, it's the tastiest of oils. Mix it in a proportion of, say, one to four with a high-rating oil to get a high-rating combination oil with superior taste.

THE HERB/SPICES FOOD GROUP FOR BEAUTIFUL SKIN

A listing of herbs and spices is of little value if you don't know which foods to use them with, so we've listed them here under the kinds of food with which they form a perfect blend-ship.

Beef
Bay leaf
Chives
Cloves
Cumin
Garlic
Marjoram
Pepper, red and black
Rosemary
Savory

Cheese
Basil
Chervil
Chives
Curry
Dill
Fennel
Garlic
Marjoram
Oregano
Sage
Thyme

Bread
Caraway
Garlic
Marjoram
Oregano
Poppy seed
Rosemary
Thyme

Fish and seafood
Chervil
Chives
Dill
Fennel
Garlic
Tarragon
Thyme

Fruit
Allspice
Anise
Cinnamon
Coriander
Cloves
Ginger
Lemon verbena
Mint
Rose geranium
Sweet cicely

Lamb
Garlic
Marjoram
Oregano
Rosemary
Thyme

Pork
Coriander
Cumin

Garlic
Ginger
Pepper, red and black
Sage
Savory
Thyme

Poultry
Garlic
Oregano
Rosemary
Sage
Savory

Salads
Basil
Borage
Burnet
Chives
Herb vinegars
Sorrel

Soups
Bay leaf
Chervil
Marjoram
Rosemary
Savory
Tarragon

II

Helping Prevent and Curb Skin Disorders

5   *Helping Prevent and Curb Acne*

Acne is a disease that strikes more than eight out of ten adolescents. It also hits middle-aged persons under stress. It is frequently one of the most distressing symptoms of the premenstrual syndrome. When one nutrient mineral, iodine, is in excess in the diet, there is nobody of either sex or in any age group who is not a candidate for acne.

An ugly disease, its symptoms are identified by an ugly name: zits. A zit can be a whitehead, a blackhead, or, in the terminology invented by dermatologist Dr. Jonathan Zizmor, a redhead. A whitehead is a small white or flesh-colored dome on your skin; a blackhead, a black dome; and a redhead, an inflamed whitehead or blackhead. All, when infected, are pimples. One zit in medical nomenclature is a comedo; more than one are comedones.

The areas of your body invaded by the zits are the face, neck, shoulders, upper chest and back. The intensity of the invasion varies. The zits may be a scattered few, no bigger than pinheads; or they may virtually overwhelm the affected area, growing to the size of small peas. Some of the zits may fill with pus—the ooze-y yellowish-white by-product of infections; others may develop into bag-like structures containing liquid, semi-liquid and even gas. The pus-filled pimples are pustules; the bag-like pimples, cysts.

"When the first serious acne patient was brought to me," Dr. Kurt W. Donsbach, a pioneering authority on the nutritional treatment of acne, remembers, "I was shocked . . . but tried desperately not to show it. . . . A young man . . . 14 years of age . . . stood before me . . . his face so covered with cysts and pustules that he refused to look at anyone . . . his back and chest a weeping mass of large open pustules. The mother told me he refused to go to school and always went to his room when any visitors came to the house. You can imagine the psychological effects on this young man!"

Acne can leave permanent scars, not only on the body but also on the psyche.

What happens when you contract acne

What you're looking at on the following page is a cross-section diagram of a cylindrical structure in the skin called a follicle.

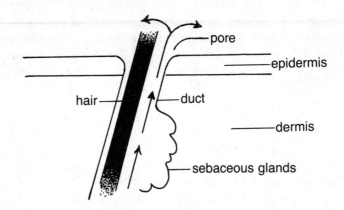

It's composed of a hair (but not always) and a duct that connects the sebaceous glands to an opening in the surface of the skin, a pore. The sebaceous glands manufacture sebum, an oily waxy substance that rises in the duct (see ascending arrows), then pours out on the skin to form a coating that prevents excess loss of water through evaporation. Sebum also helps keep the skin pliable and lubricates the hair.

Sebum has another function: to get rid of dead skin cells in the duct. When it performs that function, the skin remains healthy. When it doesn't—acne.

Here's what happens.

The cells of the inner walls of the duct, like all skin cells, are in constant regeneration: old cells die, new cells take their place. Sebum is sticky, and as it rises it pulls the dead cells from the walls, and carries them out through the pore. But when too much sebum is produced, the dead cells are drenched with the stick-um and adhere inseparably to each other and to the walls of the duct. The rising sebum can't budge them.

Now acne begins to develop. As more cells die, the walls of the duct thicken. In the narrowed duct, the sebum moves with the sluggishness of cars on a thruway where all lanes but one are closed. Faster-moving sebum fresh from the sebaceous glands impacts with the duct sebum to commingle into a dense, compact mass. When the duct narrows to such an extent that the pore closes, that mass is trapped. With no way out, and growing rapidly as the sebaceous glands continue to overproduce, the dense mass exerts pressure on the walls of the duct, ballooning them out into a dome-like structure: a whitehead. When the pore doesn't close, some of the mass extrudes, but it's so dense it can't spread. Locked in place, it's attacked by the air (oxidized), bacteria turns black, and forms an impenetrable seal over the duct. The situation now is the same as that of a closed pore. The domelike structure that results is a blackhead.

The infections caused by the mingling of sebum and bacteria transform whiteheads and blackheads into redheads, intensify the disfigurations of the disease, speed its spread throughout the affected areas, and heighten the chances of scarring and pitting. One type of bacteria associated with acne (*propionibacterium acnes*) ruptures the follicle wall and propels the infected sebum through the skin tissues, forming colonies of the disease in other follicles (called pustules near the top of them, papules somewhat lower, and abscesses around the base).

Although most adolescent victims of acne experience only one bad year, acne can begin around puberty and continue into the early twenties. After twenty-five, adolescent acne is uncommon, but several hundred thousand over-twenty-fives suffer from premenstrual-, stress-, and even sunlight-induced acne. Particularly susceptible to the latter condition (dubbed the Favre-Racouchot syndrome) are fair-skinned sun worshippers.

But whatever the trigger mechanism of acne, it begins physiologically with the overproduction of sebum. Keep that in mind. Contemporary nutritional scientists have associated it with a deficiency of vitamin A—a subject we'll discuss at length later in the chapter.

Conventional medical treatment of acne

Except for the prescription drug Accutane applied to the treatment of severe cystic acne, there is no conventional medical cure for the disease in any of its stages. (Accutane, though, has many undesirable side effects, as we shall see; and in the first two years following its approval in 1982 by the Federal Food and Drug Administration, there have been twenty reported cases of severe birth defects and twenty-four miscarriages among women using the drug during pregnancy.) The object of conventional medicine at present is to control the disease, provide cosmetic improvement, and alleviate the symptoms. No preventive program is offered because, as a distinguished panel of medical authorities have concluded, "acne cannot be prevented"—a position sharply in contrast to that of today's nutritional therapists.

Here is a review of the basics of standard medical practice in the treatment of acne. It covers the kinds of soaps and scrubs, topical drugs, antibiotics, and other therapies commonly employed.

Soaps and scrubs. Some soaps are antiseptic cleaners. Some are scrub soaps—those with abrasive action to remove undesirable surface skin. Some are both. The soaps are almost always used in conjunction with abrasive scrub cloths and other scrub (epiabrading) tools such as loofahs and the Buf-Puf. Together, they're the instruments for aggressive washing and scrubbing known as epidermabrasion. This is an exercise designed to scrape off acne debris from the outermost layer of the epidermis, the stratum corneum, while increasing blood flow to invigorate the existing surface cells and stimulate the production of new ones. Five aggressive washings a day are frequently prescribed.

Topical drugs. They're applied directly to the skin, and they're supplied as gels, lotions, creams and liquids. There are four types of topical drugs used to treat acne: peeling agents, astringents, Retin-A and moisturizers.

Peeling agents, which remove undesirable skin and loosen hardened sebum, are either exfoliants (they plane off, exfoliate, the skin), abrasives (they act as sandpaper on the skin), and benzoyl peroxide compounds, which are anti-bacterial exfoliants.

Astringents stop acne secretions by shrinking or puckering the skin.

Retin-A, a brand name of tretinoin, acts by stimulating new cell growth and helping rid the follicles of the impacted dead cells that cause acne.

Moisturizers compensate for the significant drying out of the skin caused by other topical drugs, particularly Retin-A. The much-prescribed A-hydroxy-acid "moisturizers" are not moisturizers at all but mild acids that promote the removal of undesirable dry surface skin, making room for new skin cells, which are naturally moister.

Antibiotics. The most successful in the treatment of the bacterial infections associated with acne are the tetracyclines, the erythro-mycins, and clindamycin, when taken orally. Topical antibiotics, such as phenol and chlorhydroxyyquinoline, are also employed.

Other treatments. Among them are exercise, meditation, and control of foods that, in the opinion of the doctor and the patient, aggravate the condition. For severe acne only, injections of corti-costeroids directly into the affected area, and oral dosages of Ac-cutane, are sometimes prescribed. Acne scars are treated in some cases by skin-peeling with strong acids, followed by scraping with surgical instruments. In some other cases, the scars are treated to make them indistinguishable from the rest of the skin by raising the troughs of the scars to skin level with injections under them of commercially prepared collagen, a protein found naturally in skin.

Assessment of conventional medical treatment of acne

To treat mild acne, one celebrated dermatologist prescribes, over a 30-day period, six kinds of acne-preparation soaps, three kinds of epiabrading tools, two kinds of astringents, two kinds of moisturizers, and nine kinds of peeling agents—plus aerobic exercises, relaxation exercises, meditation, and some dietary restrictions.

But no matter what combination of medical therapies are employed, pubescent acne can at best only be contained and its symptoms ameliorated, with two exceptions. Retin-A has in some cases been shown to prevent the formation of new comedones; and Accutane, as we've already indicated, has been successful in some cases in the treatment of severe cystic acne at whatever stage of life it occurs. Retin-A has also been successful in treating some mild cases of post-pubescent acne.

Here is an assessment of each of the conventional medical treatments we've already discussed, measured against its side effects and FDA standards for its effectiveness.

Soaps and scrubs assessed. Side effect: possible irritation. Effectiveness: The antiseptics in the soaps are of little or no value because they're washed off too rapidly. They and the abrasives are FDA-classified as "ineffective for the purpose intended."

Topical drugs assessed (peeling agents, astringents, Retin-A and moisturizers).

Peeling Agents. Side effects: may irritate the skin, often inducing burning, redness, swelling, dryness and itching. Those peeling agents containing the powerful irritant benzoyl peroxide may produce intense stinging and burning sensations, severe drying and reddening of the skin, and may damage the sensitive tissue around eyes, mouth, and neck. Fair-skinned acne sufferers are particularly susceptible. Effectiveness: Effective for the purpose intended, which is, practically speaking, to induce cosmetic improvement.

Astringents. Side effects: possible irritation. Effectiveness: Effective for the purpose intended, which is to provide temporary relief of the disagreeable running-sore symptom.

Retin-A. Side effects: Causes photosensitivity (increased sensitivity to light) in one out of two users, resulting in intense reddening of the skin; and may increase sensitivity to wind and cold as well. It may be irritating, particularly during the first week of use, and may induce distressing dryness, particularly in the eyes and mouth. It may raise blood-lipid (fat) levels, a condition associated with cardiovascular diseases, including heart attack. It may be toxic. Effectiveness: Retin-A may take four to six weeks to produce results, during which time it may make the affected areas look worse because of intense redness, some blistering and crusting, change of pigmentation and excessive swelling due to water retention.

Moisturizers. Side effects: A-hydroxy-acid moisturizers may cause irritation, particulary on first use. Effectiveness: Effective for the purpose intended.

Antibiotics assessed. Side effects: may irritate the gastrointestinal tract, anus, and genitals; induce diarrhea, severe dermatitis (reddening of the skin accompanied by itching), rashes and hives; and may even worsen the acne. Tetracycline destroys some vital intestinal bacteria and increases the need for vitamin C. All prescribed antibiotics decrease the absorption of vitamin A (keep that in mind) and other necessary vitamins and minerals. Effectiveness: Topical antibiotics have little or no effect on acne-associated bacteria, which are located under, not on the surface, of the skin. The value of these drugs in controlling the spread of surface infection is doubtful.

Other treatments assessed (nondrugs and drugs).

Nondrugs. Aerobic exercises, properly executed, effectively increase blood flow to all parts of the body, including the skin. That makes for a skin better fed and oxygenated, a healthier skin overall; and in that respect, aerobic exercises are helpful. But they are not a specific remedy for acne. Meditation, insofar as it's able to control stress, can weaken one trigger mechanism of the disease, but it's ineffective as a cure. Control of foods—the proper diet, supplemented if necessary—is, to nutritional scientists, the key to the acne puzzle. But conventional dermatologists, limited to striking some adverse-reaction foods from the diet while failing to add any remedial ones, do not possess the key. Their half step in the right direction, though, can be helpful. Surgery can repair the damage after the disease has struck. The techniques are safe and effective, but any single surgery is only as safe and effective as the surgeon.

Drugs. Corticosteroids are effective in treating inflammation and may ameliorate some other symptoms. The side effects, though, are some of the most alarming in the *United States Pharmacopeia.* They're summarized in the following chapter (page 50).

Accutane (isotretinoin or 13-cis retinoic acid) is chemically related to Retin-A and causes similar side effects (page 40). In addition, Accutane induces cheilitis (inflammation of the lip) in 90 percent of patients; conjunctivitis (inflammation of the membrane covering the eye) in 40 percent; disturbances of the musculoskeletal system in 16 percent; rash and temporary thinning of the hair in 10 percent; and, in about 5 percent, peeling of palms and soles, skin infections, urogenital and gastrointestinal disorders, fatigue, headache, and increased susceptibility to sunburn. In less than 1 percent of patients, among the thirteen adverse reactions reported by the manufacturer are: disseminated herpes simplex, respiratory infections, red patches on the skin, and gastrointestinal bleeding.

The manufacturer warns against the use of this drug by pregnant women, because of the possibility of major fetal abnormalities, and by nursing mothers because of the potential adverse effects on infants. The FDA has warned blood banks not to accept donations from people being treated with Accutane.

Accutane is effective in four-month, and sometimes eight-month, treatments of severe cystic acne only.

The nutritional approach to acne

This is the scenario for the onset of acne as composed by contemporary nutritional scientists.

The production of sebum from the sebaceous glands is regulated by a biochemical mechanism. When that mechanism malfunctions, overproduction occurs, and, as explained previously, the interaction of excess sebum with bacteria irritates the follicles, bringing on acne. The mechanism malfunctions when it is deficient in its principal component. The principal component is vitamin A (retinol).

Among adolescents, vitamin A entering or stored in the body is diverted from the skin to meet the demands of the body's stepped-up sex-hormone factories. Result: deficiency of vitamin A in the sebaceous glands' regulatory mechanism. Acne.

Among premenstrual women, vitamin A entering or stored in the body is diverted from the skin to meet the demands of the body's stepped-up female-hormone factories. Result: deficiency of vitamin A in the sebaceous glands' regulatory mechanism. Acne.

Among stress victims, vitamin A entering or stored in the body is diverted from the skin to meet the demands of the body's stepped-up stress-hormone factories. Result: deficiency of vitamin A in the sebaceous glands' regulatory mechanism. Acne.

One more example. Remember the Favre-Racouchot syndrome that strikes fair-skinned sun worshippers? Unchecked by dark pigmentation, the lethal rays in the sun's spectrum decimate the skin's vitamin A. Result: deficiency of vitamin A in the sebaceous glands' regulatory mechanism. Acne.

Acne is inextricably linked to vitamin-A deprivation in the skin. That has become evident not only to nutritional scientists but also to pharmaceutical researchers. Working on the premise that dosages of vitamin A large enough to compensate for the deficiencies that trigger acne would be toxic, they synthesized more than fifteen hundred vitamin A–like compounds in the last decade in a heroic quest for safe replacements. The results of their efforts to date are Retin-A and Accutane.

Nutritional scientists, on the other hand, point out that there is no danger of vitamin-A toxicity when RDA's of certain naturally occurring food biochemicals, the retinoids (carrots are loaded with them, for example), are converted by the body's intestinal cells into vitamin A. This is the safest way to bring sufficient vitamin A to the skin to help prevent acne from ever flaring up, and to damp it down in mild cases when it does.

Helping prevent and curb acne

Helping prevent acne. The first rule of prevention is: Go on and stay on your supplemented Eat for Beautiful-Skin Menus. They provide the quantity of vitamin A required to meet most people's normal needs. Then, to meet the abnormal needs during the four trigger conditions for acne—adolescence, premenstrual period, stress, and excessive exposure to sunlight—increase your daily intake of vitamin A by 5,000 to 10,000 IU's. One exception: If you're an adolescent male, add 10,000 to 15,000 IU's. Reason: the manufacture of the male hormone, testosterone, in the body steals more vitamin A from the skin than from the manufacture of the female hormones, estrogen and progesterone; and even more vitamin A is needed for sperm production. Do remember that the amounts of vitamin A *you* need to help prevent acne may be higher or lower than those suggested; or you may not need to add any vitamin A at all to your diet. Check with your doctor.

Recent research has identified close chemical relatives of vitamin A, the retinoids, as allies of vitamin A. They can also be transformed to vitamin A in the body. You can obtain additional quantities of vitamin A as retinoids by making your selections from the foods listed in the 20 Best Sources of Vitamin A, on page 145, and substituting them for other menu foods in matching food groups. For example, high vitamin A-content carrots can be substituted for any foods in the Fruit/Vegetable Food Group, page 26, when you're on our Eat for Beautiful Skin Menus or you're making up your own. You can also obtain your additional vitamin A in supplement form. Look for a fifty-fifty mixture of retinol and retinoids. It's the most effective vitamin-A product for helping prevent acne and for your general health as well.

Warning: Vitamin A (retinol) can be toxic. Consumption of more than 85,000 IU's daily over a prolonged period may result in such toxicity symptoms as headaches, profuse sweating, abdominal pain, fatigue, dizziness, vomiting, diarrhea, loss of appetite, hair loss, high blood calcium, dry skin, and brain damage. The safety limit for older children is 10,000 IU's daily, but it's prudent not to supplement a child's diet with vitamin A without your doctor's approval.

Do not take vitamin-A supplements while you're on the Pill. It raises blood levels of the vitamin, and could in effect create an overdose. Do not use vitamin-A supplements during pregnancy, either, since high blood levels of the vitamin could be harmful to the fetus. And, although there's no general proscription against vitamin-A supplements while nursing, play it safe and skip them. RDA's for pregnant women and nursing mothers are 5,000 and 6,000 IU's respectively—quantities likely to be obtainable from any healthful diet.

On the other hand, you could be taking the right amounts of vitamin A—the quantities we suggest to help prevent and curb acne—yet still be underdosing. Reason: Some substances and conditions interfere with your body's utilization of the vitamin. They include a heavy protein diet, polluted air, lengthy TV-watching, prolonged exposure to bright lights and glare, and consumption of fruit and vegetables fertilized with nitrates or treated with chlorinated pesticides. Some therapeutic drugs also induce vitamin-A underutilization, including mineral oil (a laxative); cholestyramine, a blood-cholesterol reducer more familiarly known by its brand name Questran; and, shockingly, two kinds of medications used to treat acne—antibiotics and anti-acne soaps that contain iodine or iodine compounds (Betadine, for example).

Iodine and its compounds (potassium iodide, a drug widely used to combat fungal infections, is one) are powerful inducers of acne, possibly because they block vitamin A's passage into the skin cells. "Iodine . . . is so potent an acne causer," states acne expert Dr. James E. Fulton, Jr., "that skin researchers . . . use a few drops of potassium iodide on the skin to create acne in just one week."

But iodine poses an even greater threat when consumed in foods, including one favorite of many health-conscious Americans. "Natural food enthusiasts may be disappointed to learn," comments the prestigious *Tufts University Diet and Nutrition Letter*, "that a high kelp diet can cause acne." A built-in component of that marine vegetable, iodine occurs just as naturally in a wide variety of foods.

To help prevent acne (if you're prone to it), eat the following high-iodine foods sparingly; and if you're subject to acne flare-ups, don't eat them at all: asparagus, beef liver, broccoli, clams, corn, crab,

hamburger, kelp, onions (white), potato chips, salt (seasoned, io-
dized, sun-evaporated and uniodized), stew meat, squid, tortilla
chips, turkey and wheat germ. Even with that abstinence you're
likely to obtain your RDA of iodine from your supplemented Eat
for Beautiful Skin Menus.

Bromine and bromides, chemical relatives to iodine, should also
be ingested sparingly. The chief culprits here are some cough
medicines and some vegetable oils. Bromine and bromides as potential acne-inducers are newcomers on the scene, and the statistics are just being fed into the computer banks. In the meantime,
read labels, and address your questions to the American Association of Dermatology, 820 Davis Street, Evanston, Illinois 60201.

On the other hand, except for about one in a hundred acne
sufferers, foods traditionally associated with acne no longer are.
They include chocolate, french fries, nuts, "greasy platters," colas,
pizzas and some seafoods. But for overall beautiful skin and good
health, it's a bright idea to keep these foods, except seafood, out of
most of your meals.

And let's shatter another myth: Abstinence from sexual activity,
solitary or otherwise, has nothing to do with preventing acne.

Helping curb acne. "There have been notable successes with retinol [vitamin A] ... in cases of acne," reports science writer John
O'Rourk. "One combination of diet and stress treatment is ...
claimed to be 100 percent successful by Dr. Kenneth Flandermeyer.... And Dr. Flandermeyer's years of research and wide
practice ... in dermatology makes his testimony impressive."

Nutritional therapy for acne, which should only be instituted
under your doctor's care, is based on adding sufficient quantity of
vitamin A to the diet. This helps repair the damage done by deficiency of the vitamin and restores the optimal amount of vitamin
A in the skin system. Just how much vitamin A is sufficient for
these purposes depends largely on the severity of the disease. But
one thing is certain: Whatever quantity of vitamin A is prescribed,
it will work most effectively if it's added to an RDA diet, such as
the diet supplied by your supplemented Eat for Beautiful Skin
Menus. On that diet, to which 5,000 to 10,000 IU's of vitamin A
(10,000 to 15,000 if you're an adolescent male) have been added
daily, there is some evidence that mild cases of acne may be
helped, particularly when accompanied by conventional hygienic
measures.

Dr. Michael Colgan recommends that "if you get recurrent acne," increase, in addition to vitamin A, potassium and zinc by 30 milligrams each, and "eat eggs, onions and garlic for sulfur," possibly to increase the efficiency of the vitamin. Hint: "To avoid garlic/onion breath," advises Francine Prince, the nation's leading authority on cooking for better health, "mince or chop—never use a garlic press, and use the natural breath sweetener, parsley."

6 *Helping Prevent and Curb Psoriasis*

Unsightly, uncomfortable, mentally distressing, psoriasis afflicts up to eight million Americans, mostly adults between the ages of twenty-five and fifty. Although the disease leaves no scars and is not contagious, malignant or life-threatening, more than $1.5 billion is poured out yearly by its victims in attempts, almost always in vain, to wipe out its symptoms. Described by physicians as "tenacious, chronic, stubborn, recurring," psoriasis is among the ugliest common diseases known to medical science.

It starts (usually in young adulthood, but any age can be a starting age) with the eruption of small, dull red spots covered with dry whitish-gray or silvery scales that conceal tiny bleeding points. The spots erupt in patches which, in a short time, merge into larger patches, called plaques, that look like the shells of oysters, if you can imagine bright-red oysters; or resemble just as fiery hued mica, a glass-like mineral composed of many thin layers. The former plaques are called ostraceous; the later, micaceous.

Itching may occur, but not characteristically; and the malady is so otherwise unaccompanied by overt symptoms of ill health that the National Psoriasis Foundation calls it the "disease of healthy people." This is basically an affliction that affronts the eye of the victim and the beholder, its unsightly appearance heightened sometimes by discolored and pitted fingernails that may crack and split, and even separate from the fingers.

Psoriasis can strike any spot on the body, but the areas in which the eruptions are most likely to occur are: the scalp, ears, elbows, hands, nails, lower back and knees.

What happens when you contract psoriasis

Simply stated: The control mechanism for skin cell production goes wild.

Normally, skin cells are born in the lowest level of the epidermis, rise to the surface, die, flake off, and are replaced by new skin cells which, in their turn, have ascended from below. The time it takes for this to happen is called the "turnover rate"—and in healthy skin it's about 28 days. But when the control mechanism for skin cell production goes wild, the turnover rate is speeded up by a factor of 10. New cells zip to the surface every 2.8 days. But it still takes 28 days for the surface cells to die. Result: pile ups. They take the forms of the ostraceous and micaceous plaques of psoriasis. Large quantities of blood piped to the surface of the skin to feed a 1,000-percent increase in cell population turns them flaming red.

The malfunction of the control mechanism for skin cell production, and the consequent psoriatic flare-ups can be triggered at a specific site by an injury (cut, burn, surgical incision) or by excessive pressure (when the pressure is on hands swinging a golf culb, the variety of psoriasis is called Koebner's phenomenon). Widespread attacks can be set off by stress, excess physical exertion, and certain illnesses including diabetes, strep throat, flu and other infections of the upper respiratory tract. Arthritis in particular could bring on psoriasis (one out of every twenty arthritics are psoriatics), and so could some gene lurking in your chromosomes until the time is right to express itself (psoriasis runs in the family of one out of ten victims). Sunburn can induce the malfunction.

But how do these trigger mechanisms—all so different—work? What do they have in common? Nutritional scientists believe they all deplete the skin's store of vitamin A and of at least one essential fatty acid. We'll look into that in depth later on in this chapter.

Conventional medical treatment of psoriasis

Although, as you know from Tere Ingram's story, there may be a successful nutritional approach to what one physician calls "the heartbreak of psoriasis," all a doctor will promise, as a matter of standard practice, is to try to keep the disease under control and provide some relief from its symptoms. He can keep that promise in five different ways: with coal-tar derivatives, with corticosteroids, with sunlight and ultraviolet light, with PUVA, and with anti-metabolites. Here are thumbnail sketches of each of this quintet of therapies:

Coal-tar derivatives are complex organic chemicals derived from a by-product of coal. They have been employed in the treatment of skin disorders since the 1920s when they were hailed as wonder drugs. They act to soften scaly skin and reduce itching and peeling. Some coal-tar derivatives are mixed with antiseptics, astringents and moisturizers, which act as they do in anti-acne preparations (page 37). Coal-tar-derivative preparations are supplied as creams, emollients, gels, lotions, ointments, shampoos and soap.

Corticosteroids are, in nature, members of a family of steroid hormones manufactured in the outer part of the adrenal gland, the cortex (hence the name, corticosteroids). In the pharmaceutical industry, corticosteroids are those natural products, or synthetic look-alikes and derivatives, or new compounds chemically related to the originals. Applied topically as creams and ointments, or injected directly into the psoriasis sores, corticosteroids act to reduce the severity of the symptoms.

Sunlight and unltraviolet light. Dermatologist Dr. Jerome M. Aronberg, although realizing that psoriasis sufferers are reluctant to sunbathe in the presence of others, recommends full body exposure to sunlight "until pink" to control the disease. Sometimes ultraviolet light is prescribed instead of sunlight.

PUVA involves the use of the drug, *p*soralen, which is activated by *u*ltraviolet *A* light (string the italicized letters together and you get PUVA). It acts to control scaling and flare-ups.

Antimetabolites are drugs developed to treat cancer by disrupting the metabolic processes of cancer cells, halting growth, creating malfunctions, and sometimes killing the cells. These drugs attack psoriatic cells in the same manner.

Assessment of conventional medical treatment of psoriasis

In a recalcitrant case of psoriasis, a dermatologist may use all five standard therapies. In addition to attempting to keep the disease from worsening and to decrease the severity of the symptoms, he may hope to hasten remission. In this disease, remission occurs frequently without medical aid, but recurs just as frequently despite medical aid.

Here is an assessment of the five standard medical treatments for psoriasis, measured against their side effects and FDA standards of effectiveness.

Coal-tar derivatives assessed. Side effects: Overall rating is "possibly unsafe." Coal-tar derivatives are known carcinogens. Effectiveness: Not enough data to make a judgment. (If that lifts your eyebrows in view of these preparations' more-than-sixty years of life in the marketplace, here's the explanation. Back in the 1920s, when these drugs made their debut, there was no FDA; and FDA requirements for safety and effectiveness are not retroactive.)

The common additives to psoriasis coal-tar-derivative preparations rate as follows. (*Unsafe* means "unsafe for the specific medical use," and *ineffective* means "ineffective for the purpose intended"; *safe* and *effective* means the opposites). Benzalkonium, an antiseptic: *unsafe, ineffective*. Alcohol, an astringent: *safe, effective*. Salicylic acid, a moisturizing agent and skin softener: not enough data to make a judgment on safety; *ineffective*.

Corticosteroids assessed. Side effects: Prolonged topical use may lead to acnelike eruptions, dermatitis, atrophy (wasting away) of the skin, high blood pressure, burning sensations, dryness, infections of the follicles, irritation, loss of skin pigments, prickly heat (sticky, extremely small blisters in the folds of the skin), striae (raised streaks of a different texture and color from the skin), and excessive hair growth, including facial hair on women as well as men.

Prolonged use by injection into the sores may lead to hypoglycemia (low blood sugar) and diabetes (high blood sugar) due to increased demands for insulin; muscle wasting and weakness, due to breakdown of proteins; bone fractures and other skeletal injuries, due to loss of bone tissue; higher incidence of viral, bacterial, and fungal infections, due to destruction of white cells; ulcers, due to greater secretion of gastric juices; and abnormal mental states including euphoria (feeling exhilaratingly happy when there's nothing to feel happy about), irritability when there's no reason to be irritable, and hyperkinesia (a compulsive need to be in motion). Sudden termination of treatment after prolonged high dosages can be fatal.

Effectiveness: Initial successes in reducing scaling and controlling flare-ups can be dramatic. But over a long period, the disease is likely to return to its original intensity or even worsen. Recurrences after remissions occur with greater frequency than when coal-tar derivatives are used.

Sunlight and ultraviolet light assessed. Side effects: Condition may be worsened by overexposure, and almost certainly by sunburn. Overexposure may also induce other skin diseases, including cancer. Efficiency: Insufficient data to make a judgment. But some dermatologists report excellent results, particularly when used with coal-tar derivatives, in reducing redness, promoting skin healing and suppressing the disease.

PUVA assessed. Side effects: premature skin aging, skin cancer, cataract formation, burns. Psoralen may be a carcinogen. A recently developed chemical relative of psoralen, trisoralen, (trioxdalen), claimed to be more effective, has not been approved by the FDA for the treatment of psoriasis. Effectiveness: Insufficient data to make a judgment, but some good short-term results have been reported. One dermatologist, in fact, claims a symptom-removal success rate of 88 percent. A recent review of medical skin problems in a national woman's magazine calls PUVA "the newest, simplest, and most effective treatment for severe psoriasis that does not respond to other methods."

Antimetabolites assessed. Methotrexate (formerly known as A-Methopterin) is a typical antimetabolite, prescribed mainly for the management of breast cancer. The manufacturer prints this warning in capital letters in its package insert (a brochure describing the product):

DEATHS HAVE BEEN REPORTED WITH THE USE OF METHOTREXATE IN THE TREATMENT OF PSORIASIS. METHOTREXATE SHOULD BE RESTRICTED TO SEVERE, RECALCITRANT, DISABLING PSORIASIS WHICH IS NOT ADEQUATELY RESPONSIVE TO OTHER FORMS OF THERAPY. . . .METHOTREXATE MUST BE USED ONLY BY PHYSICIANS EXPERIENCED IN ANTIMETABOLITE CHEMOTHERAPY.

Side effects (this is a selection): skin rashes with itching, welts, acne, loss of skin pigmentation, skin discoloration due to the infiltration of blood into the skin, boils, dilation of small blood vessels, hair loss, chills, fever, headaches, fatigue, nausea, vomiting, diarrhea, loss of appetite, anemia, menstrual disorders, convulsions, brain damage, possible infections due to adverse effect on the immune system, and paralysis.

Effectiveness: The manufacturer claims the drug is effective for the purpose intended. The drug is FDA-approved for effectiveness and safety.

The nutritional approach to psoriasis

This is the scenario for the onset of psoriasis as composed by contemporary nutritional scientists.

The production of skin cells is controlled by a biochemical mechanism. A malfunction of the mechanism causes overproduction, bringing on psoriasis. The malfunction occurs when there is a deficiency in the principal component of the mechanism. That principal component is vitamin A.

Every trigger mechanism of psoriasis, through its own biological pathways, depletes the skin of vitamin A. As a matter of fact, the need for vitamin A in the treatment of psoriasis has been so firmly established that conventional medical scientists, wary of the vitamin's alleged toxicity, have been experimenting with "safer" synthetic A-like replacements. At the University of Michigan Medical School, they seem to have found one, etretinate, that works, but its side effects can elevate blood lipids and cholesterol into the red-alert zone, and the patient in effect could be swapping psoriasis for heart attack.

Sound like a rerun of the scenario for acne? It is—so far. But a big difference has been written in: another component now shares the principle role with vitamin A. It's a fatty acid.

A fatty acid may be saturated, mono-unsaturated or polyunsaturated. Saturated fatty acids are found in animal fats; two vegetable fats, palm and coconut; and commerically hydrogenated fats, such as Crisco and margarine. Olive and peanut oils contain mono-unsaturated fatty acids. Polyunsaturated fatty acids abound in the oils of the vegetable and marine kingdoms.

Among the polyunsaturated fatty acids are the essential fatty acids, the EFA's. Like vitamins they are vital, in minute quantities, for the healthy functioning of the body. They "not only act like a vitamin," writes pioneer nutritionist, Dr. John Yudkin, "but for some time they were referred to by some research workers as vitamin F." Thought just a few years ago to be just three, the number of EFA's is now six. One of those six is arachidonic acid. It's the fatty acid that shares the directorship of the skin-cell-production mechanism with vitamin A.

Among the recent breakthroughs in our knowledge of the chemistry of the human body is the discovery of how arachidonic acts in skin cell production. With the aid of other body chemicals, it changes (metabolizes) into a biochemical called PGE_1,—a hormone-like substance. (A hormone gives the chemical commands that activate cells, tissues, organs, and the body itself.) PGE_1 gives commands to the skin-cell production mechanism.

How PGE_1 shares its command function with vitamin A is at this time unknown. But one thing is certain: Normal PGE_1 and vitamin

A levels in the skin are the keys to normal skin-cell production. And arachidonic acid and vitamin A in optimal quantities in your Menus are the keys to normal levels of PGE$_1$ and vitamin A in the skin. Those levels may help prevent psoriasis, and, in mild cases, curb it.

Helping prevent and curb psoriasis

Helping prevent psoriasis. Again, the first rule of prevention is: Go on and stay on your supplemented Eat for Beautiful Skin Menus. They provide vitamin A and retinoids in sufficient quantity to meet the normal requirements of most people. But during any extended abnormal condition that could trigger psoriasis (see list, page 48), the addition of 5,000 to 10,000 IU's of vitamin A to compensate for the loss of that vitamin in the skin system may help prevent the onset of the disease. In the preceding chapter, you learned how to obtain that additional vitamin A from retinoids in your food.

Your Eat for Beautiful Skin Menus also supply you with about the amount of arachidonic acid consumed by non-psoriatic Americans—about 100 milligrams a day. In any of the trigger conditions in which arachidonic-acid depletion may occur, it's a preventive-wise idea to add another 50 milligrams of this EFA to your diet. Do it by making selections of arachidonic-rich foods from the chart on page 160, and substituting each food selected for one in the same Food Group in your Menus. Hint: An extremely small amount of walnut oil—about a tenth of an ounce—replacing, say, corn oil in your salad dressing, can supply the additional 50 milligrams of arachidonic acid you may require.

All these psoriasis-preventive suggestions should be followed only on the advice of your doctor.

Helping curb psoriasis. Tere helped curb her mother's psoriasis. But scientists will tell you that what Tere did was not necessarily the result of the nutritional approach. The disease may have gone into remission by itself. They'll also tell you that what worked for Tere's mother may not work for anybody else. All that is true, which emphasizes once again that should you consider nutritional therapy as an alternative to the conventional treatment of any skin disorder including psoriasis, talk it over with your doctor before you do anything; and undertake the treatment only under his care.

What Tere did was place her mother on a basic RDA diet—your

supplemented Eat for Beautiful Skin Menus—augmented with 10,000 IU's of vitamin A as a supplement. The menus were also modified to supply an additional 100 milligrams of arachidonic acid daily from a selection of arachidonic acid-rich foods. Should your doctor approve this therapy in principle, you can obtain the amounts of vitamin A he prescribes from foods as well as from a supplement. Each vitamin A– and arachidonic acid–rich food should replace a food in a matching Food Group in your Menus. There's a list of vitamin A–rich foods on page 145, and of arachidonic acid–rich foods on page 160. Remember also that retinoids are allies of vitamin A in helping maintain healthy skin. Retinoid-rich foods—including yellow, orange and deep-green fruits and vegetables—should be eaten daily.

If you get recurrent mild patches of psoriasis, Dr. Michael Colgan recommends taking, in addition to augmented quantities of vitamin A, 40 milligrams of vitamin B_6 and 45 milligrams of zinc daily; plus eggs, onions, and garlic for their high sulfur content. These additional nutrients probably help vitamin A and arachidonic acid undo the damage caused by the disease (which is to say, undo the damage caused by vitamin-A and arachidonic-acid deficiencies in the skin system) and maintain the health of your skin.

7 *Helping Prevent and Curb Eczema*

Itching of such fierce intensity that it can wreck sleep, make a shambles of your daily routine, and provoke uncontrollable scratching characterizes severe eczema. In gradations of intensity, from mild to monstrous, eczema (atopic dermatitis), strikes millions of Americans at age two months, continues to age four years, goes into retreat until adolescence, then hangs on until about fifty. It is a disease of explosive flare-ups and merciful calms. But the flare-ups at their scratch-compulsion worst can wrack the brain and torture the emotions.

A raised rash and swelling are the usual early signs of the disease. Small blisters (vesicles) form, then as time goes on, progressively ooze, crust, scale, and shape into patches of thick, dark, dry skin. Eczema can hit anywhere on the body, but the preferred target regions are the face, neck, scalp, the upper back, the bends of the knees and elbows and the other folds of the body. The more widespread the disease, the more severe the itching.

What happens when you contract eczema

Specifically, conventional medical science has no idea how this disease is caused. Some trigger mechanisms have been identified, but there doesn't seem to be any common denominator; and in many cases, eczema breaks out with no apparent trigger mechanism. But generally, medical thinkers realize that some things must happen when you contract eczema: Something must happen to the nerves to cause the itching; something must happen to the skin cells to cause the pustules; something else must happen to the skin cells to cause the ultimate dryness—and all three somethings must be related.

Certainly, that's no explanation. But it's a clue—and that's the clue that unlocked the secret of eczema to the nutritional scientists, as we shall see later in this chapter.

Conventional medical treatment of eczema

Standard medical practice offers no cure for eczema, and no preventive program. It does hold out hope, though, of lessening the severity of the symptoms. The usual course of medical treatment consists of:

Treating oozing pustules with an astringent to stop secretions by shrinking or puckering the skin. Compresses soaked with Burow's solution are the usual means of application.

Alleviating dryness with moisturizers and bath preparations.

Countering itching —when it's mild, with oatmeal preparations; when it's severe, with coal-tar preparations and corticosteroids, separately or together; and when it's widespread, with antihistamines.

Assessment of conventional medical treatment of eczema

The treatments are measured here against the side effects and the FDA standards for effectiveness.

For treating oozing pustules, the most commonly used preparation is Burow's solution. Side effects of its active ingredient, aluminum acetate: Overall rating, unsafe or potentially unsafe for the specific medical use. Effectiveness: Ineffective or potentially ineffective for the purpose intended. Nonaluminum acetate astringents, although they may sting and irritate, are safe and effective, and provide some temporary relief.

For alleviating dryness, the side effects of moisturizers and bath preparations are limited to possible stinging and irritation; and they are effective for temporary relief of the symptoms.

For countering itching, oatmeal preparations have no adverse side effects, and they are effective for temporary relief in mild cases. Coal-tar preparations are neither safe nor effective (see page 49). Corticosteroids induce a long list of severely adverse side effects (see page 50) but are effective for short periods for the purpose intended. Both coal-tar derivatives and corticosteroids have been known to worsen eczema in some patients.

Antihistamines are employed as anti-itching agents on the supposition that the itching is, in whole or part, caused by the action of histamines, substances produced by the body to counter the

action of alien chemicals, in this case some of the chemicals produced by the diseased skin cells. A typical antihistamine (a drug
that's antagonistic to the histamine) employed to alleviate widespread eczema-induced itching is Antihistamine Cream. Its two
active ingredients, methapyriline HC1 and pyrilamine, have no significant adverse side effects. They are judged safe for the specific
medical use, and effective in supplying temporary relief—which,
for sufferers from the unrelenting severity of widespread eczema
itch, could mean a few hours' decent sleep.

For treating infections, antibiotics induce numerous adverse
side effects (see page 40) but are judged safe for the specific medical use and effective in controlling most of the bacterial infections
associated with the disease.

The nutritional approach to eczema

The clues held by nutritional scientists attempting to solve the
mystery of eczema consisted of three interrelated symptoms: a
specific kind of damage to the skin, intense itching and severe skin
dryness. Here's how they used those clues to piece together the
broad outlines of a nutritional theory of the cause of eczema,
which appears to stand up under some clinical tests.

The specific kind of damage to the skin—the vesicles, the crusts,
the scales—bear a family resemblance to the flare-ups of psoriasis.
That disease is caused by a malfunctioning of the control mechanism of skin-cell production, induced by deficiencies in vitamin A
and arachidonic acid, an essential fatty acid (EFA). It seemed likely
that the visual symptoms of eczema could be caused by similar
deficiencies. Experiments corroborated the hypothesis, except
that not one EFA was involved but four, with the most-needed role
going to gamma-linolenic acid. (The other three EFA's involved are
linoleic acid, linolenic acid and arachidonic acid.)

Deficiency of EFA's hooked in with the severe dryness symptom.
Deprivation of EFA's had not only produced that symptom in laboratory animals, but the visual symptoms of eczema as well.

That left only the severe itching to be accounted for. The intensity was too fierce to be caused by histamines alone; besides, although antihistamines lessen the intensity of the itching, they
don't eliminate it. Something else had to be at work, and that
something caused nerve ends to send out abnormal signals—
scratch-me signals—to the skin. Deficiency of vitamins of the B-

complex, nutritional scientists know, could do that. Moreover, B-complex deficiencies were also known to cause skin dryness, scaling and sores—tightly tying the B-vitamin complex to the eczema syndrome.

What the interpretation of the clue of the three interrelated symptoms added up to was this: A triple nutritional deficiency—in vitamin A, B-complex vitamins and EFA's—is a possible cause of eczema.

Helping prevent and curb eczema

Within the last few years positive reports on stopping eczema before it starts and checking it afterwards (when it's mild) have appeared in scientific publications here and abroad. Even the conservative *Tufts University Diet & Nutrition Letter* published the results of a 1984 study providing evidence that a diet leading to EFA deficiency can worsen eczema, and of another study in the same year that reported beneficial effects of gamma-linolenic acid in the treatment of the disease.

The following program for helping prevent and curb eczema is based on experimental and clinical evidence appearing in the scientific literature. Nutritional allowances are suggested, but since each person is different, it's wise to check yours with your doctor.

Helping prevent eczema. Preventive nutritional therapy is based on keeping optimal quantities of vitamin A, vitamins of the B complex and EFA's in the skin system at all times. The first rule of prevention, therefore, is, as always: Go on and stay on the supplemented Eat for Beautiful Skin Menus. They provide all the anti-eczema nutrients in sufficient quantities to meet the normal requirements of most people.

However, there are conditions that diminish the skin system's store of these nutrients and may lead to outbreaks of eczema. Among these conditions are: a family history of the disease; skin contact with soaps, detergents, synthetic clothing, or wool; stress; and excessively hot or cold weather. Not all these conditions induce eczema in all people; and most people are not likely to contract the disease under any of those conditions. But to stay on the safe side, augmenting your diet with anti-eczema nutrients under your doctor's supervision under these conditions is a good idea. Not too much is known about all the trigger conditions for eczema, so it's also a good idea to check with friends and relatives about other conditions that cause their flare-ups, and to augment your diet with anti-eczema nutrients when you're exposed to *those* conditions as well.

Here is a suggested eczema-prevention formula for use under conditions that may induce eczema by nutrient depletion in some people:

Vitamin A	5,000 to 10,000 IU's daily
Vitamin B complex	One "B-50" product daily
EFA's	About 3,500 milligrams daily

Here's a guide to obtaining each of these nutrients in the right quantities:

Vitamin A can be obtained from retinoid-rich foods (see chart, page 145), substituting any of those foods for a food in a matching Food Group in Your Eat for Beautiful Skin Menus; as well as from a vitamin-A supplement.

Vitamin B, in the quantity required, can only be obtained from a supplement. To acquire 100 milligrams of vitamin B_1 from its No. 1 food source, for example, you would have to consume about two and a half pounds of soybeans a day. You would need about twenty-five to thirty pounds of food daily to get your full quota of eczema-preventive B's.

In nature, however, B-complex vitamins co-exist with other nutrients that contribute to the B's efficiency in the body. For that reason, it's advisable when you're exposed to conditions that may trigger eczema to up your intake of vitamine B-rich foods. You'll find the 20 best sources of each of the B-complex vitamins listed on pages 146 to 152. Substitute your choice of each of these foods for a food in a matching Food Group in Your Eat for Beautiful Skin Menus.

Warning: When you're adding vitamins of the B complex to your diet, keep in mind that some, and sometimes many of these vitamins can be rendered useless—just as you discovered that much of your vitamin A intake could be rendered useless—by substances and conditions that interfere with your body's utilization of these vitamins. Here's the catalog:

Physical or emotional stress can deplete vitamins B_1, B_3, and folic acid (one reason why stress can lead to eczema). Air pollution is an enemy of vitamin B_1. A high-carbohydrate diet, such as those favored by many reducing-diet doctors, can knock out vitamin B_3. Food additives, particularly nitrites, sulfites (nitrites are in wursts, bacon, ham; sulfites are in dried fruits), and baking soda, can destroy vitamin B_1. Raw egg whites and choline (in lecithin) are biotin antagonists. And alcoholic beverages deplete your skin cells of vitamins B_1, B_3, and folic acid.

But the greatest enemies of vitamins of the B-complex—and such great enemies of all vitamins that Dr. Daphne A. Roe, professor of nutritional science at Cornell University, calls them "antivitamins"—are some of our therapeutic drugs. An up-to-date list of those drugs appears on the following page.

ANTI-VITAMIN-B-COMPLEX DRUGS

Drugs	**Vitamins Depleted**
Antibiotics	B_1, B_2, B_3, B_6 (penicilamine) B_{12} (neomycin, chloramphenicol), biotin, inositol
Anticonvulsants (including diphenyl hydantoin and primidone)	B_6, B_{12}, folic acid
Antimalarials (including pyrimethamine)	B_6, B_{12}, folic acid
Antituberculars (including isoniazid, INH, PAS, and cycloserine)	B_3, B_6, B_{12}, folic acid
Aspirin and aspirin substitutes	B_{12}
Codeine (a cough-medicine compound)	B_{12}
Cortisone (see corticosteroids, page 49)	B_6
Hydralizone (A hypertensive: a drug that lowers blood pressure)	B_6

Levodopa (used to treat Parkinson's disease)	B_6
Methotrexate (used to treat cancer and severe psoriasis)	Folic acid
Mineral oil (a laxative)	Inositol
Oral contraceptives	B_2, B_6, B_{12}, folic acid
Phenobarbital	B_6, B_{12}, folic acid

What can you do in practical terms about vitamin-B depletion? Go on and stay on your supplemented Eat for Beautiful Skin Menus. They contain no vitamin-B depletants, and they help you compensate for the loss of vitamin B due to the depletants in your environment and life-style. But the supplemented menus do not protect you against anti-vitamin-B drugs. If you have to take any of those drugs, ask your doctor to prescribe a compensatory dosage of the depleted B's.

EFA's can be obtained from foods; and you'll find the best sources listed on pages 159–160. Substitute each food you select for a food in a matching Food Group in the Eat for Beautiful Skin Menus.

Gamma-linolenic acid, which plays a major role in eczema prevention, is manufactured by the body. It is not present in any food in appreciable quantities except in the oil of the evening primrose, a night-blooming flower grown in this country and in Canada and England. It is available in health food stores.

Warning: There are certain EFA's that really aren't EFA's at all and can block the action of gamma-linolenic acid. These are the *trans*-EFA's, made up of the same chemical components as the true EFA's—the *cis*-EFA's—but shaped differently. The *trans*-EFAs, shaped like wide horseshoes, literally surround the more compact straight-line *cis*-EFA's and take them out of the action.

So, it's prudent when you're exposed to conditions or substances that could induce eczema to eliminate *trans*-EFA's from your diet, and to minimize them at other times. Foods containing *trans*-EFAs include animal fats, butter, margarine (soft, soft/tub, diet), mayonnaise, nondairy creams and toppings, shortenings, commercially processed vegetable oils, and all products made from them (especially candies, baked goods, fried foods, salads, and desserts). Examine labels and remember, when the label reads "partially hydrogenated vegetable fats," it means *trans*-EFA fats.

Helping curb eczema. For recurrent mild eczema, additional quantities of vitamin A, B-complex vitamins and EFA's, in connection with conventional hygienic measures, have been recommended by nutritional therapists. Dr. Michael Colgan adds iodine as well, perhaps as an aid to the body's better utilization of the other nutrients. What quantities of anti-eczema nutrients are right for you should be determined by your doctor, who is indispensable in the treatment of this disease. Our research suggests that an eczema-prevention formula (page 59) may be helpful in curbing eczema.

Do remember that nutrient augmentation is useful only when it's applied to a nutrient-rich diet—the kind of diet you enjoy with your supplemented Eat for Beautiful Skin Menus.

8 *Helping Prevent and Curb Herpes*

One type of herpes simplex, one of the more common diseases known to the human race, a perennial, with a medical pedigree dating back to ancient Rome, is usually a minor irritant as diseases go. The other type, with as antique a heritage, but for millenia not a commonplace ailment, has erupted in the United States in the last decade into a raging epidemic that has already claimed 20,000,000 victims, with more than 750,000 predicted by Federal authorities for the year ahead. This type of herpes is severely painful, physically embarrassing, can lead to cancer and fetal fatalities, and carries with it a social stigma. The mild type is herpes simplex I. It appears mostly as the common cold sore. The harsh type is herpes simplex II. It attacks the genitals.

Herpes simplex I, as almost all of us know, usually begins to create problems as a burning, tingling or itching sensation on a slightly reddened site on the upper lip. Pass a fingertip lightly over the affected area and you'll feel, even though you can't see, a slight bump. In a day or two, suddenly that bump breaks out into blisters, some as small as pinheads, some as wide as quarters, and some in assorted sizes in between. Then, over the course of the next few days, the blisters burst, the open sores harden, yellowish crusts develop and fall off, and the lip is left as unmarred as it was before. But as lenient as herpes simplex I is most of the times, on occasions it can be cruel. It can plague the face and other parts of the body with painful zitlike outbreaks; exacerbate nerve-related dermatitis; and scar the cornea of the eye, impairing vision. In newborns, if passed on by the mother, it can damage the brain; and in infants, it can cause a type of blood poisoning, viremia, that can be fatal.

Herpes simplex II is transmitted during sexual intercourse. The disease appears first as severe pain or itching and swelling in the genital regions. Vulva, vagina, cervix, anus, and penis are affected, as well as the thighs and buttocks. In about a week, small painful sores tender to the touch appear; and in the male, they crust much like cold sores. Fever, a sore throat, and a general flu-like feeling complete the syndrome. The herpes sores, which heal like those of herpes simplex I without medical care, leave no scars. The symptoms of the disease are gone in about three weeks.

But not the disease.

Once you have contracted either type of herpes, you're likely to have it for life. After the initial attack, the disease lies dormant, but may break out intermittently thereafter. Recurrent cold sores may be no more than a nuisance, fairly well concealed by medicated masking preparations, but repeat flare-ups of genital herpes can be as wracking as the first-time attack, and dangerous. The mortality/deformation rate among infants born of mothers actively infected with herpes simplex II is one out of four. The presence of active herpes simplex II virus in the female genitals increase the risk of cervical cancer by 800 percent. (Cervical refers to cervix, the opening of the uterus, also known as the womb.) The effect on the emotional lives of the victims can be heartbreaking.

To those who suffer twelve to sixteen attacks per year, genital herpes, according to science writer Phillip M. Boffey, "disrupts . . . marital and social relations, and drives some to suicide." Perceived by a large segment of mature Americans as the wages of sexual freedom—*Time* magazine cover-storied the disease as "The Scarlet Letter of Our Generation"—genital herpes is to many infected by it a more severe psychological and social affliction than it is a physical one. "Genital herpes," writes Dr. Cory SerVaas, one of the nation's leaders in the war against the disease, "often has [such] a devastating psychological effect on its victims [that they] say they 'feel like lepers.'"

What happens when you contract herpes

A virus is raw DNA—the basic genetic stuff that directs the reproduction, identity, and growth of living things—in a protein capsule. But a virus can't reproduce itself. Not yet really living (if reproduction is a criterion of life), the virus only becomes alive when it invades a living cell, links itself with *that* cell's DNA, and uses *that* DNA to reproduce itself—profusely. In science-fiction what happens could be called "The Invasion of the Cell Snatchers." In science fact, it's a viral infection.

Herpes is a viral infection. It's a strange one because of a behavior pattern no one has yet fathomed. After the initial attack is over, the herpes virus takes up residence in the body's nerve roots and stays there. Nothing happens. Nothing may ever happen. But pull certain triggers—get into a stressful situation, expose yourself to strong sunlight, let yourself come down with a respiratory infection, manage a gastrointestinal upset, or involve yourself in some other abnormal state—and then the virus strikes out from its base and attacks. When the attack is over, the virus returns to its base. And waits.

Conventional medical treatment of herpes

There is no prevention or cure for herpes from conventional medicine. But there are palliatives. A palliative is a medicine that may bring relief of symptoms without attacking the underlying cause of the disease.

For the cold sores and related zit-like blemishes of herpes simplex I, there are a number of palliatives of the kinds we've already met in this book for the treatment of other skin conditions—astringents, antiseptics, and analgesics. A doctor may prescribe them with this sound advice: Don't touch the sores, don't play with them, don't pick at them, don't get them wet, and don't band-aid them. Ignore those prohibitions and you could extend healing time.

The astringents give you the feeling that the sores have been contained, that they won't ooze endlessly. The antiseptics help prevent secondary infections that can turn blisters into painful, slow-healing blemishes. The analgesics are pain-relievers. But basically, if you keep your hands off the sores, even without medical aid, the virus will usually go away in a week or ten days—from the skin, that is.

For genital herpes, conventional medicine offers, at best, similar symptom alleviators; and, at worst, a hodgepodge of desperation remedies. One genital-herpes victim described her medical treatment to Dr. SerVaas: "I contracted genital herpes when I was very young—sixteen and in love. I was treated ... with silver nitrate, gamma globulin, smallpox vaccine, soda baths and many things without success. In the ten years I was under treatment, I had attacks every four months. My doctor really didn't know what to do."

But currently there is great hope among medical experts that broad gains in the treatment of genital herpes lie in the not-too-distant future. "The number of companies attempting to develop vaccines," reports the University of Chicago's Dr. Bernard Roizman, a leading authority on herpes, "is increasing every year." A herpes vaccine is a medication that uses dead virus or weakened live virus to stimulate the production in the body of certain antibodies, members of the immune system that recognize the herpes virus and destroy it. Such a vaccine was developed successfully in Germany some years ago, but is banned in this country because its major side effect is cancer. Target date for an American-made FDA-approved herpes vaccine in 1989, provided what some investigators regard as formidable obstacles (safety, effectiveness) can be overcome.

Hope for a faster breakthrough resides in the medical profession's faith in the pharmaceutical industry. "The number of companies investing money in developing [antiherpes] drugs," says Dr. Roizman, "is phenomenal." The one drug thus far developed that could knock out the herpes virus is carcinogenic and not approved for use. But a new drug, FDA-approved in 1983, works on the same principle—the disruption of the genetic structure of the invader—as one class of sometimes successful anti-cancer drugs. This new drug, Zovirax (acyclovir), may be the prototype of a family of more effective antiherpes drugs.

Assessment of conventional medical treatment of herpes

Doctors can choose from the well-stocked pharmacy of astringents, antiseptics and analgesics, most of which work for the purpose intended with a minimum of adverse side effects. (The list of these drugs is much too lengthy to be included here, but since no drug is side-effect-free, it's prudent and your legal right to request from your doctor a description of the possible side effects of any drug, prescription or over-the-counter, that he recommends. Several excellent all-about-drugs reference books are listed under Recommended Reading on page 166.)

The adverse side effects of the only drug used to treat the disease and not the symptoms, Zovirax, are surprisingly moderate as reported by the manufacturer. They are: discomfort in application, transient burning and stinging, mild pain, rash, pruritis (severe itching) and vulvitis (inflammation of the vulva, the opening to the vagina). So far as the effectiveness of the drug is concerned, Dr. Cory SerVaas, reported:

"We did research on Zovirax and came to the conclusion that, at $20 an ounce, it is quite expensive for the use to which it can be put. The FDA recommends that Zovirax ointment be prescribed only for patients with first-time infections. It has no benefit for anything except relieving the pain of the first outbreak . . . and may help reduce the length.

"Burroughs Wellcome Company, which developed Zovirax and is marketing the ointment, said that the medication is not being promoted for use in recurring episodes, where it has no effect. People who have already had one attack of herpes are wasting their time and money using Zovirax to treat subsequent attacks."

For first-time genital herpes infections, the manufacturer claims for both topical and intravenous administrations of the drug, "significant effects ... in elimination of the [herpes] virus from the lesions [sores] and in reduction of healing time."

The nutritional approach to herpes

The herpes simplex viruses I and II belong to a group of herpes viruses responsible for a number of maladies including chicken pox, shingles (a notoriously ugly and painful skin condition), mononucleosis, Bell's palsy (a certain kind of paralysis of the face) and Ménière's disease (a balance and hearing disorder). In 1952, a strain of herpes virus causing brain infections in mice and humans was subjected by investigators at the University of Southern California (USC) to experimental treatment with naturally occurring amino acids. A routine experiment, this was to be the basis, in later years and with different investigators, for the development of the first nutritional therapy for a viral infection.

Amino acids are the building blocks of life; one way or another, they enter into every living biochemical reaction. Of the twenty-two amino acids necessary for human biochemistry, fourteen are manufactured in the body. The other eight, called the essential amino acids, come to us in our food. The USC investigators discovered that one of the essential amino acids inhibited the growth of the herpes virus. That amino acid is lysine. The discovery lay neglected in the scientific archives for a dozen years.

Then, Dr. Robert Tankersley, studying a herpes virus at the Medical College of Virginia, came across the report of the USC experiment, reran it, and corroborated the findings. Attempting to discover whether other amino acids would act like lysine, he made a serendipitous discovery. No other amino acid duplicated lysine's inhibitory effect on the herpes virus, but one amino acid did just the opposite. Arginine, a nonessential amino acid, stimulated the reproduction of the virus. Tankersley's work added up to this:

When a herpes virus is in a nutrient solution containing more arginine than lysine, it can be activated, and it thrives. But when it's in a nutrient solution containing more lysine than arginine, it cannot be activated, and if it has already been activated, it stops reproducing. Backup research at medical centers in this country and Israel supported Dr. Tankersley's findings. The arginine-lysine connection with the herpes virus had been established. In the laboratory.

But no practicing physician was willing to break with standard vaccine/drug therapy to test the effects of these naturally occurring amino acids (they're in supermarket foods) on herpes patients. It wasn't until 1974, a decade after Dr. Tankersley's breakthrough, that three courageous medical investigators decided to put Dr. Tankersley's findings to a clinical test. Dr. Arthur Norins, head of the dermatology department of the Indiana School of Medicine, and his colleagues Dr. Christopher Kagan and Dr. Richard Griffith treated herpes simplex I and II patients with a diet low in arginine, supplemented with lysine.

The results: In hundreds of cases, there were no recurrent flare-ups—the test of success in the treatment of herpes. Relief of symptoms was rapid and dramatic as well. "Patients start lysine, and the thing they remark about it is that they forget they had the lesions [sores] in a matter of hours," Dr. Griffith testifies. "The pain is gone.... It works better on genital than on labial," he adds. (Labial refers here to the lips.) Dr. Norins says the arginine-lysine treatment has a success ratio of 9 out of 10. "The other 10 percent who were having the most severe problems," he admits, "had not been helped."

While supporting clinical evidence for this first nutritional therapy for a viral infection is abundant, arginine-lysine treatment is not standard medical practice. Detractors point to a study conducted at the University of Miami, Florida, that was unable to detect improvement due to lysine in herpes conditions. However, the investigators did not establish the presence of a positive lysine-to-arginine ratio in the body's amino-acid pool, casting doubts on the validity of their conclusions.

Helping prevent and curb herpes

The recommendations that follow are based mainly on the work of the Norin-Kagan-Griffith team, and the independent findings of Dr. Barbara North and the Colgan Institute of Nutritional Science, San Diego. These recommendations are, like all others in this book, subject to your doctor's review. But bear in mind that while the new generation of nutritional doctors are likely to prescribe arginine-lysine therapy, conventional doctors are not. One thing is certain: There are no adverse side effects from adding lysine to your diet (it's an essential amino acid, necessary for your body's well-being) or subtracting arginine from it (your body normally manufactures all the arginine you need).

Helping prevent herpes. Deficiencies of nutrients in the average American diet over the last decade includes lysine. That, perhaps, makes sexual liberation a secondary cause of the spread of genital herpes. So step one in the prevention of herpes simplex of both kinds is to be sure your diet contains more lysine than arginine. It does when you go on and stay on the Eat for Beautiful Skin Menus.

If you're exposed to herpes—and remember, investigators are certain both types are spread from one person to another by contact, and are not certain either type can be spread any other way—then add 500 milligrams of lysine daily to your Eat for Beautiful Skin Menus. You can obtain this quota by modifying your Menus with selections from the chart of The 20 Best Sources of Lysine, page 161, substituting the foods you choose for foods in matching Food Groups in your Menus; or you can take the amino acid as an L-lysine supplement.

The L- is important because that variety of lysine is more potent than the D- or the DL- varieties. D- and L- forms of a chemical compound are made up of the same components, but each form is structured so that it's the mirror image of the other. In nature, one of the mirror images possesses greater biological activity than the other. In this case, it's the L-. DL- represents a mixture of the two forms. (D- stands for *dextro*, right; L- for *levo*, left.)

If you're between herpes flare-ups, 500 milligrams of lysine a day is usually prescribed by doctors who treat patients with the arginine-lysine therapy.

But not even 6,000 milligrams a day will prevent herpes, Dr. Griffith warns, if your diet is laden with high-arginine foods, such as chocolate, nuts, peanut butter, seeds, jello and cereals. To be sure to establish a strongly positive lysine-to-arginine ratio in your body, eliminate or minimize the foods listed in the chart of *The 20 Highest Arginine-Containing Foods* on the following page.

THE 20 HIGHEST ARGININE-CONTAINING FOODS

How to use this chart: If you've been exposed to herpes, or if you're between herpes attacks or undergoing a herpes attack, eliminate these foods from your diet.

	Excess arginine over lysine in milligrams, uncooked
Hazel nuts, ½ cup	2,250
Brazil nuts, ½ cup	2,210
Peanuts, ½ cup	2,060
Walnuts, ½ cup	810
Almond, ½ cup	710
Cocoa powder, ½ cup	650
Peanut butter, 2 tablespoons	510
Sesame seeds, ½ cup	450
Cashews, ½ cup	420
Carob powder, ½ cup	310
Coconut, ½ cup	290
Pistachio nuts, ½ cup	240
Buckwheat flour, ½ cup	230
Chick-peas, ½ cup	210
Rice, brown, ½ cup	190
Pecans, ½ cup	180
Whole-wheat bread, 4 slices	160
Oatmeal, cooked, ½ cup	130
Raisins, ½ cup	130
Sunflower seeds, ½ cup	120

Also avoid chocolate, jello, and all breakfast cereals, which seem to boost the effects of arginine.

Helping curb herpes. Dr. Cory SerVaas, assessing the results of a survey conducted by her among physicians nation-wide who prescribe lysine in the treatment of herpes simplex I and II, reports "very positive and exciting results" when patients took 1,500 to 3,000 milligrams of L-lysine supplement in three doses daily. "In addition," she writes, "all of the physicians with whom we spoke insisted that decreasing the intake of arginine was equally important in creating a bad environment for the herpes virus." That can be done by eliminating The 20 Highest Arginine-Containing Foods on the previous page. It's also wise, according to Dr. Michael Colgan, to eliminate citrus juices, which seem to exacerbate herpes sores.

Dr. SerVaas is convinced that herpes is prevented and curbed most efficiently when L-lysine supplements augment a high-lysine diet; and she has placed the resources of *The Saturday Evening Post*, of which she is the editor-in-chief, behind the development of such a diet. Her two most notable achievements in that respect thus far have been publicizing the recent development of a high-lysine corn by Purdue University's Dr. Edwin Mertz and Dr. Oliver Nelson (corn, an inexpensive, high-fiber staple, is normally virtually devoid of lysine); and commissioning the nation's best-selling author on cooking for better health, Francine Prince, to create a "gourmet high-lysine cuisine."

For information on how to obtain copies of *The Saturday Evening Post* containing features on these projects, as well as on the nation's most complete ongoing coverage of developments in arginine-lysine therapy, write: *The Saturday Evening Post Society*, Division of the Benjamin Franklin Literary & Medical Society, 1100 Waterway Boulevard, Indianapolis, Indiana 46202.

9 *Helping Prevent and Curb Premature Skin Aging*

Would you like to know how old you are? *Really* are? Make the following test. You can do it in seconds.

Place a watch with a seconds indicator in front of you. Hold out one of your hands, fingers straight, palms downward. Pinch the back of the hand in the region midway between the knuckles and the wrist. Draw up the skin as far as it can go. Let go. Take a seconds reading on your watch. When the pinched skin has returned to normal, take another reading. Note the elapsed time:

Up to 2 seconds means your "real" age is under 45.

Up to 20 seconds means your "real" age is 45 to 65.

Up to 50 seconds means your "real" age is 65 to 75.

More than 50 seconds means you're actually older than 75.

Now compare your "real" age—your biological age—with the age on your nearest birthday—your chronological age. If your biological age is greater than your chronological age, you're aging prematurely.

Although all organ systems in the body age at different rates (your nervous system remains 90 percent efficient at age 75, for example, while your heart's pumping efficiency drops to 40 percent), the skin is the key marker of the aging of the body as a whole. That's why, if you haven't been exposed to excess sunlight—it's a deadly enemy of the skin, aging it rapidly and irreversibly—the pinch test reflects your real age.

The pinch test tells you at the same time how much your skin has aged. But it's the eye test that tells you how it's aged. Aged skin is arid, rough, horny, blemished. It's leathery. It's laugh-lined, and worry-lined, and whisper-lined (those vertical lines around the mouth). It's wrinkled. It has crow's feet. It's color-drained, drab, littered with dull brown age spots. It droops, sags, hangs shapelessly. Look at the skin on your aged face, and, remembering the skin of your youth, it looks as if you were wearing a mask. But you can't take it off.

Aging is sad. But premature aging is sadder. Aging is inevitable.

But premature aging is not. Not for your skin, and not for your whole body, when you follow some simple nutritional guidelines. Stop premature aging that way, and, if you had been gaining an extra quarter year of age for each passing year, as most American women do, then next year you'll begin to look younger than most women of your age, four years from now a year younger, and ten years from now, when it counts, two and a half years younger.

What happens when your skin ages

Dr. Roy L. Walford, world-renowned research scientist at the University of California Los Angeles (UCLA) Medical School, is the nation's leading authority on aging. This is his explanation of what happens when your skin ages: "The wrinkles, dryness and other changes in the skin ... whose disguise occupy so many pages of *Vogue* and *Glamour* ... are due to thinning of the superficial layer of the epidermis, deterioration of the tiny skin glands, and damage to the connective tissue (collagen and elastic fibers) deeper down. . . . [These] connective tissue become stiffer and chemically immobilized with age."

This means that there are less new cells—so the skin no longer looks fresh and rosy; less natural moisturizing agents—so the skin no longer looks shower-glistening; and less and less resiliency— so the skin no longer bounces back when you smile or frown or wrinkle your nose, and the lines of your emotions are sculptured into your flesh permanently.

Rounded out with textbook details, that's the way conventional medicine sees the skin aging process. It's an accurate description as far as it goes. It can go further with the answers to why does the skin age? and why does it age prematurely? Nutritional scientists have those answers, as we shall see later in this chapter.

Conventional medical treatment of premature skin aging

Doctors treat diseases; and they don't recognize premature aging as a disease unless it's acute—like when an 11-year-old girl looks like a sixty-year-old (there *is* such a disease: progenia). As a consequence, there is no medical textbook program for the prevention or curbing of premature skin aging. But one well known dermatologist recently claimed not only to curb aging skin but also to rejuvenate it.

Writing in collaboration with Sharon Sabin, Dr. Jonathan Zizmor states: "There is a patented formula you apply to your skin that is truly antiaging. Available by prescription, it can be used not only to reverse the complexion's ravaged appearance but also to prevent skin from ever getting old looking." The "patented formula" is Retin-A, an anti-acne drug we've already met. "In effect," the Dr. Zizmor-Sabin team continues, "Retin-A can turn back the clock for skin and return it to a more youthful condition. . . ."

The drug is applied twice a day, or every other day (if the patient can't adjust easily to the irritation), starting with the weakest formulation, a gel mixed with an equal amount of cold cream, and progressing to stronger formulations—a cream and then a liquid, undiluted—over a course of several months.

Assessment of conventional medical treatment of premature skin aging

A selection of the adverse side effects of Retin-A, the "anti-aging drug," appears on page 40. Although the drug is FDA-approved for the treatment of acne, it is not for the treatment of aged skin.

The nutritional approach to premature skin aging

Of the many extraordinary achievements of the nutritional science revolution of our times, ranking near the top or at the top is the first biological/nutritional explanation of aging and premature aging. Classic in its simplicity, it weaves together hundreds of apparently unrelated research and clinical results into a cohesive two-part pattern. It sees aging biologically as the deterioration of three interlinked body systems: the DNA, the histo-compatibility complex and the immune system. It sees premature aging as the accelerated deterioration of those systems as a result of nutrient deficiencies.

What follows is a capsule description of that pattern. It's a pattern that supplies the basis for treating and curbing all premature aging, including premature skin aging.

The pattern starts with a biological paradox. Each day we're the same, and yet we're different. We're the same because the genetic structure in our cells, the DNA, is designed to trigger each of our cells (60 trillion of them) to replace themselves as they wear out with identical cells. We're different because, past puberty, the DNA itself begins to wear out, and it begins to make mistakes; small ones, but the new cells are no longer exactly identical with the cells they replace. Imperceptible from day to day, but perceptible from one year to another, the changes in the cells, and in the stuff between them which the DNA also controls, change us. The muscles stiffen, the hair greys, the skin loses its bloom. We age.

The histocompatibility complex stands watch for alien invaders of the body (viruses, bacteria, pollutants, cancer cells, oxidants, others). Think of it as a military defense early warning system, but immeasurably more complex, more sensitive, more efficient. The function of the histocompatibility complex is to spot alien invaders and alert the immune system to seek and destroy. In youth, the performance of the complex can be flawless. But as the DNA makes mistakes, replacement cells in the complex also develop flaws. They fail to recognize some invaders, which, with no resistance against them, ravage the body. They fail, also, to recognize the new imperfect copies of our body cells as our own cells, mistake them for invaders, signal for their destruction, and turn the immune system on ourselves. In these ways we age, too.

The immune system also suffers as time goes on. With each new blunder of the DNA, change by change, the fighting cells of our body's formidable defense network, particularly the crack T-cells, decline in number, mobility and potency. By age seventy, the immune system's battle effectiveness is only 10 percent of what it was at age twenty. As our defenses against invaders crumble, infectious diseases, allergens, cancers and toxins devastate our bodies. That also ages us.

That's normal aging.

Premature aging is abnormal aging. It's a disease—the most widespread degenerative disease of our time, says Dr. Michael Colgan. It's caused when the DNA, the histocompatibility complex and the immune system are damaged, hastening the development of age-accelerated flaws. The damage comes from oxidants— those savagely destructive chemicals—produced in the body in such massive waves that they overwhelm our antioxidant defense. But had that defense been at full strength, not only would it not have been overwhelmed, but it also would have destroyed the attacking oxidants. The antioxidant defense is at full strength when it contains the right nutrients in the right amounts.

At bottom, premature aging is a nutrient-deficiency disease. It can be prevented and curbed nutritionally.

Helping prevent and curb premature aging skin

The body's antioxidant defense protects every part of the body including the skin. It's composed of the following nutrients: vitamins A, C, E, B_5, and B_6; the minerals selenium and zinc; nucleic acids (the components of DNA and RNA); cholesterol; and the nonessential amino acid, cysteine.

They act as a team, directly counterattacking the oxidants, and they help the histocompatibility complex manufacture particularly powerful anti-oxidants, the SOD's (superoxide dismutases). SOD's can be obtained as supplements, but whether SOD's in that form can be useful to the body has not yet been determined.

Earlier in this chapter, we quoted a well-known dermatologist's claim that "there is a patented formula you apply to your skin that is truly antiaging . . . Retin-A."

There *is* a formula, but it's not patented; it's natural. You don't apply it to your skin, because aging is not a local blemish; it's systemic involving whole-body systems. It's not anti-aging—nothing can stop the aging process—but it *is* anti-premature aging. And it's not Retin-A; it's a formula supplying the right amounts of nutrients in the anti-oxidant team.

Remember once again that the recommended nutrient quantities represent a consensus of numbers preferred by nutritional scientists. But *you* are not a consensus; and the numbers could be on target for you, or off the mark. Consult your doctor about what nutrients in what amounts are right for you.

Helping prevent premature skin aging. Under normal circumstances your supplemented Eat for Beautiful Skin Menus supply the right nutrients in the right amounts to help prevent premature skin aging (and premature aging of the rest of the body as well)—the complete formula.

But some of the ingredients of the formula must be augmented if you're subjected to any of the following premature-aging conditions that can sharply increase the production of oxidants or sharply decrease the body's utilization of members of the anti-oxidant team. These conditions are: mental or physical stress, illness, cigarette smoke (your own or other people's), oral contraceptives, prolonged exposure to sunlight or ultraviolet light, food additives, X rays or other radiation, excess alcohol, industrial toxins, many therapeutic drugs (see index), pollutants and high-decibel sound including rock-and-roll.

Here is a suggested nutritional formula to help prevent premature skin aging for use under premature-aging conditions in conjunction with a high-nutrient-content diet—such as provided by your supplemented Eat for Beautiful Skin Menus—under the supervision of your doctor:

Vitamin A, 6,000 I.U.'s.
Vitamin B_5, 50 mg.
Vitamin B_6, 50 mg.
Vitamin C, 500 mg.
Vitamin E, 300 IU's
Selenium, 50 mcg.
Zinc, 15 mg.

The only practical way to obtain these nutrients in the suggested quantities is with supplements. However, foods rich in these nutrients are likely to contain other nutrients which improve the efficiency of the formula; so it's a good idea when you're subjected to premature-aging conditions to include in your Eat for Beautiful Skin Menus foods high in anti-premature-aging nutrients. Consult the charts of The 20 Best Sources of Selected Essential Nutrients in the Appendix, and substitute each of your selections for a food in a matching Food Group in your Menus.

Two of the members of the anti-oxidant team, nucleic acids and cysteine, do not need to be augmented. The reasons:

The Eat for Beautiful Skin Menus are rich in foods high in nucleic acids including sardines (the best source), herring, tuna and anchovies among canned fish; bass, flounder, halibut, salmon, scrod and trout among fresh fish; liver and other organ meats; and yeast, spinach and oatmeal.

However, Dr. Robert C. Atkins, who finds nucleic acids "useful" in the treatment of aging skin, acne and many degenerative diseases, sometimes starts treatment with a supplement of 1,200 milligrams of RNA daily. (RNA, very closely related to DNA, transfers DNA instructions to the protein-producing factory in the cell, the ribosome.) Dr. Benjamin Frank, the discoverer of the anti-oxidant properties of nucleic acids, although recommending increased consumption of nucleic-acid-rich foods, treats his patients for aging as well as degenerative diseases with between 30 and 1,300 milligrams of RNA daily, several times a week. Sandy Shaw of the well known (Durk) Pearson-Shaw nutritional team, includes an occasional 1,000-milligram RNA supplement in her personal life-extension (anti-aging) programs. But Drs. Atkins and Frank and Ms. Shaw apparently use RNA supplements to augment an average American diet—which can use all the help it gets—and not the optimal-nutrition Eat for Beautiful Skin diet.

Similarly, the 1,000 to 2,000 milligrams of cysteine on the Pearson-Shaw experimental "life-extension" (anti-aging) supplement formulation is meant to be added to the average American diet, which may be low in cysteine, and not to the Eat for Beautiful Skin Menus, which are rich in such high-cysteine foods as eggs, meat and cheese. Our diet also contains two to three times as much vitamin C as cysteine, which prevents cysteine oxidizing in the body to cystine, another amino acid which could help form bladder and kidney stones. Moreover, cysteine is a nonessential acid—it's manufactured by the body—and the Eat for Beautiful Skin Menus provide all the nutrients in the right amounts for its optimal production.

Helping to curb premature skin aging. Cross-linkages are a major contributor to aging skin. Think of cross-linkages this way. Picture a shift of workers, shoulder to shoulder, facing an assembly line. Their hands are free, and they work with suppleness and fluidity. Enter terrorists. They handcuff the workers together, left hands to left hands, right hands to right hands, so the hands cross in front of their bodies. Cross-linked now, the workers' hands are immobile, rigid, useless. And the lock on the handcuffs is unbreakable.

In the skin (and throughout the rest of the body), the workers are strands of collagen. The terrorists, oxidants. The handcuffs, the cross-linking process itself. The collagen, that once provided flexibility and resilience to the skin, now becomes inelastic, hard, tough and wrinkled—and so does the skin. The cross-linkages are irreversible.

But while you can't undo the cross-linkages, you can slow down the rate of future cross-linkages—and the rate of all other skin- (and body-) aging processes—to normal. The formula is the same as for preventing premature aging skin, except the numbers are higher.

Here is the revised nutritional formula to help curb any additional premature skin aging, for use with high-nutrient-content diet, such as provided by your supplemented Eat for Beautiful Skin Menus, under the supervision of your doctor:

Vitamin A: 10,000 IU's
Vitamin B$_5$: 75 mg.
Vitamin B$_6$: 75 mg.
Vitamin C: 1,000 mg.
Vitamin E: 400 IU'S
Selenium: 50 mcg.
Zinc: 15 mg.

Use supplements, and enrich your Eat for Beautiful Skin Menus with foods rich in the formula nutrients, just as you did in helping prevent premature skin aging (page 77).

10 *Helping Prevent and Curb Skin Cancer*

Of the hundreds of types of cancers that the National Cancer Institute tells us will strike one out of three Americans by age seventy-four, skin cancer is the most common. If you're fair-skinned, blond, and blue-eyed, you're most susceptible. (But if you're Black, Oriental, American Indian, or Hispanic, you have little to worry about.) After age fifty, your vulnerability increases. Some skin cancers can kill.

It's not hard to recognize cancer growths on your skin. One type starts as a tiny knot-like lump protruding from the surface. It's pearly and translucent. It grows quite slowly, then becomes a sore discharging pus. This type of skin cancer is called basal-cell carcinoma. (A carcinoma is a cancer that starts in the skin or mucous membranes.)

Another type of skin cancer first appears as a small raised patch. It's probably darker than the skin, may be red, and it's usually hard. Nothing happens for months, perhaps years, then it starts to grow. It becomes a pus-filled sore crusted with scales. It's particularly ugly on the lower lip, which it appears to favor. This is squamous-cell carcinoma. (Squamous means scaly.)

The final type of skin cancer usually begins when a color change occurs in or around a pigmented mole. The mole itself could turn colors from reddish to blue-black; or a patch of red or other color could encircle its base. Then, rapidly, the mole darkens, grows into a pus-filled sore and bleeds. This is malignant melanoma. (A melanoma is a mole colored with the dark skin-and-hair pigment melanin. A malignant melanoma is one that's cancerous.)

Metastasis, which is the appearance of cancer in parts of the body not connected with the original tumor, is rare in basal cell carcinoma—almost never happens; but this type of cancer can eat deeply into bordering tissue. Squamous-cell carcinoma metastasizes frequently; the favorite target areas are the ears and backs of the hands. Malignant melanoma can metastasize to vital organs swiftly; and it's the chief cause of death from skin cancer.

What happens when you contract skin cancer

We've talked up to now about biochemical mechanisms that control the birth, growth and activity of the cells. Actually, they're submechanisms. The basic mechanism, which determines *their* structure and function, is a double helix (think of two spiral staircases intertwined) composed of about 1,000,000 units. Each unit is different. Each unit is a gene. These genes, by directing the production of the submechanisms, manage what a cell looks like, what it does, and what its relations are to the other cells in the body. Normal active genes, providing none of the submechanisms malfunction, produce normal active cells—like healthy, beautiful skin cells.

But not all the million genes in the double helix (the DNA strands) are active; and some of the normal active ones could be transformed into abnormal ones. Bring into the cell the destructive chemicals spewed out by stress, mental or physical; or bring in certain viruses; or pollutants in air, water and food; or radiation: X-ray, cancer-therapeutic, military or industrial; or excess of sunlight or ultraviolet light; or a pharmacy of therapeutic drugs; or the fumes of cigarettes, cigars and pipe tobacco—and normal genes can turn into potential killers; and some genes, always potential killers, but dormant, can be stimulated into action. These are the oncogenes. They turn normal cells into cancer cells.

Cancer cells are malignant (tending or threatening to produce death) because they are unlike normal cells in these respects:

• They reproduce at high speed; and, with no built-in mechanism to stop them, can build a colony that can go on growing forever. That mass of alien cells, existing for itself alone (all other cells in the body are interlinked for the common good), is the symbol of the disease—the tumor. ("Onco" means tumor, and "oncogene" means a gene that produces a tumor.)

• They break down the cement between cells (the collagen) that holds the body together, literally causing the body to fall apart, making it prone to degenerative diseases and infections.

• They invade, take over, and destroy healthy tissues and organs all over the body, striking through metastasis at regions remote from the original site of the tumor.

• And finally, cancer cells are malignant because the pain they can bring—excruciating, unremitting, torturous, so severe that sometimes even the most merciful narcotics are powerless against it—can hasten death.

Molecular biologists (scientists who study genes), like Dr. Robert Weinberg at the Massachusetts Institute of Technology in Cambridge, have identified some oncogenes; others, like Dr. Mitchell Goldfarb at the Columbia Presbyterian Hospital in New York, are on the track of what happens when an oncogene is activated— what biochemical processes occur that create the Jekyll-Hyde transformation of the cell. Assessing the prospects of understanding the basic biochemistry of oncogenes based on accomplishments of biochemists so far, *Nature*, one of the world's foremost scientific weeklies, commented editorially in 1983 that "for the first time, there is a chance of getting to the bottom of the phenomenon of cancer."

Conventional medical treatment of skin cancer

Prevention is, as a practical matter, limited by physicians to an early-warning-signal watch. You are advised to be alert to any skin change that does not revert to normal swiftly; and for any change in a mole. On spotting a condition-red signal, you're instructed to see your doctor fast; and, because malignant melanoma is one of the swiftest striking and deadliest of all cancers, when you spot a change in a mole, see your doctor within the hour. A biopsy (a microscopic examination of an extremely small section of the affected area) will or will not, with a good degree of certainty, reveal the presence of a malignancy.

The much-publicized nutritional cancer-prevention program— the anti-cancer diet—proposed recently by the National Cancer Institute and the National Academy of Science's Committee on Diet, Nutrition and Cancer, advises the population, in effect, to follow the Federal Dietary Guidelines for Americans: avoid overweight, eat less fat, eat more fiber, cut down on salt and sugar, drink in moderation, abstain from oversmoking, and consume a variety of foods to obtain your RDA's (Recommended Daily Allowances of nutrients). This is sound advice for maintaining good health in general (your Eat for Beautiful Skin Menus incorporate much of the Federal Dietary Guidelines), and good health in general can help cut down the incidence of all diseases including cancer.

*So far as treating existing cancer, including skin cancer, conven
tional medicine offers three types of therapy: surgery, radiation and
chemotherapy.* They're administered separately or in combina
tions.

Surgery involves the removal of the tumor and often the adjoining
tissue and lymph node. (Think of a lymph node as a combined
garbage-disposal and manufacturing plant. It disposes of bacteria
and cellular debris from tissue fluid; it manufactures lymphocytes,
white blood cells, front-line troops of the body's security [im-
mune] system that devour viruses, bacteria and other alien invaders including cancer cells. The lymph nodes are part of a
body-wide circulatory system much like the blood's and connected with the blood's. Cancer cells entering a lymph node could
easily be transported via the linked circulatory systems to every
part of the body—metastasis. This is why when a tumor is removed, the nearby lymph node is removed as well.)

Radiation from X rays, radium and radioactive cobalt pour lethal
invisible energy into targeted cancer zones. The doses are massive.
(The unit of radiation is a rad. A diagnostic dental X ray generates
1 rad. The typical cancer treatment dosage begins at 4,000 rads.)
Although employed primarily as postsurgical treatment, radiation is also employed to shrink tumors prior to surgery, and is
sometimes used independently of surgery, by itself or with chemotherapy.

Chemotherapy (the word is synthesized from "chemicals" and
"therapy"), which was developed in the forties and spread into
wide use in the sixties, has become in the eighties, according to a
recent authoritative review of cancer therapy, "the leading weapon
for increasing the number of patients who can be cured of cancer."
Chemotherapy is based on the use of chemical poisons that kill
cancer cells faster than they kill normal cells.

There are four major classes of chemotherapeutic agents for the
treatment of skin cancer (they're also administered for other types
of cancer). Each class attacks the cancer cell in a different way.
Treating a patient, a doctor may use one drug from a class or more
than one; or he may mix drugs from several or all the classes on
the theory that if the cancer cell can't be killed one way, it can be
killed another. Here's how the four major classes attack cancer:

Antimetabolites play havoc with the cancer cell's metabolism, shut down growth, and may eventually kill the cell. Examples: methotrexate (you've already met it as an antipsoriatic agent, page 51) is designated to fight a form of malignant melanoma (as well as many types of non-skin cancer); Efudix (fluorouracil) is a cream or solution administered topically to sun- or radiation-induced basal-cell carcinomas.

Alkylating agents, originally based on the powerful military chemical mustard gas, disrupts the basic genetic structure (the DNA and RNA) of the cancer cell, slowing down characteristic rapid reproduction or killing the cell. Example: BiCNU (carmustine) is employed against some malignant melanomas (as well as other types of cancer).

Antibiotics act much the same way as alkylating agents. Example: Blenoxane (bleomycin) is used against sqamous cell-carcinomas.

DTC Dome (dacarbazine) can be regarded as a class of drugs with, up to now, only one member. It acts like an alkylating agent, but is not related to that class chemically. Its targets are malignant melanomas.

Assessment of conventional medical treatment of skin cancer

Although cure rates of cancer have become suspect in recent years (one reason: many tumors diagnosed as malignant were never malignant in the first place), traditional medicine's skin-cancer cure rate is good to excellent. (A cancer cure is defined by the medical profession as a remission lasting five years.) Both basal-cell and squamous-cell carcinomas when caught early have close to a 100-percent cure rate. The cure rate of nonmetastasized malignant melanomas is about 60 percent; of metastasized, percentage figures aren't available, but the verdict is "poor."

But even when a cure is effective, the side effects are harrowing. Surgery can create disfigurement, sometimes spread the disease, and induce the now taken-for-granted traumas, mental and physical, accompanying any major invasion of the body in an operating room. Radiation (remember the 4,000-rad dosages) can bring on new cancers, and bring about radiation sickness which includes among its symptoms: severe pain, hemorrhages, anemia, loss of hair, and the breakdown of the immune system, leading to infectious diseases. It can speed up the appearance of old age by leathering the skin, and it can burn away years from a patient's life. It can leave a heritage to the newborn: deformities, among which is cancer.

But the most punishing side effects in the treatment of cancer—perhaps in the treatment of any disease since doctors a century or so ago immersed cholera patients in tubs of boiling water—arise from the expanding use of chemotherapy. The powerful cytoxics (drugs that poison all cells, not just cancer cells) devastate patients immediately after each intensive therapy session with severe nausea and vomiting, and with debilitating illnesses. Then hair falls out, diarrhea attacks, the appetite vanishes, and the blood no longer clots normally. The nervous system is violated. The sperm count plummets. The blood turns anemic. The immune system is ravaged, and illnesses that people ordinarily throw off become killers. New cancers erupt. The final side effect can be death.

Specific anti-skin-cancer drugs sometimes follow that general pattern: methotrexate, for example (you met it on page 51). More often, though, the side effects are not as adverse. Take Efudex, an antimetabolite that, administered as a topical cream or solution, can cure sun-induced skin cancer in about twelve weeks. Its side effects include: pain, severe itching, burning sensation on the skin, running sores, scaling, swelling, dermatitis, darkened skin, scarring, tenderness, sensitivity to light, anemia, and the decline of the immune system, making the body vulnerable to infectious diseases.

The overall failure rate of chemotherapy is three out of four. Cancer cells are now developing immunities to the drugs.

The nutritional approach to skin cancer

. . . is based on two simple new ways of looking at the disease.

One. Cancer—and this is a mind-boggling concept—can be normal. In a sense. Maryann Napoli, summing up our present knowledge of cancer for Medical Consumers and Health Care Information, Inc., explains:

"Many cancer researchers believe that our bodies are constantly forming cells of a cancerous nature, but most of the time they are discarded by our incredibly efficient immune system." P. B. Medawar, Nobel prize-winning biologist, says that everyone probably gets cancer thousands of times, even millions of times, during a life-span, but the cancers are destroyed by the immune system before they can grow large enough to be detected.

A basic strategy, then, in the war against cancer should be to strengthen the immune system. A potent immune system can also snuff out those viruses, and even some bacteria, that otherwise would invade normal cells and set off the cancer-transformation process. Nutritional scientists claim they can strengthen the immune system with the right nutrients in the right amounts.

Two. Cancer—and this is an equally startling concept—can be caused by innocent things. In a sense. "We know now," writes Dr. Michael Colgan, one of the world's foremost nutritional scientists, "that cancers are caused by exposure to what used to be thought of as harmless substances." He parades before his readers fruit, vegetables, meat, fowl, fish and grains—now laden with pesticides; suits, dresses, hats, gloves, lingerie—now made from polyvinyl chloride; homes and trailers—now insulated with urea foam; and virtually all the everyday products of our society—now tainted by the more than 2,300 suspected carcinogens identified by Federal agencies.

Among the innocents that cause cancer are even substances that are supposed to make us well. Dr. Colgan again: "Many, many drugs are carcinogenic, from the once common analgesic phenacetin to the synthetic hormone diethylstilbesterol (DES). . . . Everything from contraceptive pills to the common antibiotics are suspected of causing cancer. . . . Some of the anticancer drugs *cause* cancer, the disease they are meant to correct . . . The 1,470 pages of the *American Medical Association Drug Evaluations Handbook* read like a horror story."

Add one more group of innocents: working, loving, bringing up a family, playing, commuting, shopping, vacationing, driving, in short, living in the U.S.A. in the '80's—now, for many of us, burdened with stress, one of the deadliest of carcinogens.

These carcinogens work by producing a horde of marauding chemical fragments in the body. These are the oxidants. By a myriad of chemical pathways, they transform some of the normal biochemicals of the body into molecular terrorists that break through the cell's defenses and liberate the oncogenes. But the oxidants can only bring about that transformation when the body's antioxidant system is weak.

Another basic strategy, then, in the war against cancer should be to strengthen our natural antioxidant system. Some nutritional scientists claim they can do it with the right nutrients in the right amounts.

With the two strategies combined—strengthening the immune system and strengthening the antioxidant system—you may prevent cancer. Dr. Colgan goes even further and proclaims in a chapter head of one of his books: "YOU *CAN* PREVENT CANCER" (emphasis ours).

But can you *curb existing* cancer nutritionally? One eminent scientist, recipient of a Nobel Prize in chemistry, submits that it has been done. He's Dr. Linus Pauling. We'll review his claims in the latter part of the next section.

Helping prevent and curb skin cancer

Dr. Colgan again: "The mass of [positive] findings about nutrient effects against cancer is surprising. All these strong preventive effects have been found with single nutrients. . . . No one investigator has tested the effects of a complete vitamin and mineral supplement."

Your supplemented Eat for Beautiful Skin Menus not only supply Colgan's "complete vitamin and mineral supplement," but also provide RDA's of all essential nutrients, the indispensable base for good health, and *all* the single nutrients found to have strong positive cancer-preventive effects. Those nutrients, as you can expect, fall into two groups: The anti-oxidants which you've met in the preceding chapter: vitamins A, C, E, B_5 and B_6; the minerals selenium and zinc; nucleic acids (the components of DNA and RNA); and the nonessential amino acid cysteine. And the immune system boosters: vitamin C and the other vitamins of the B complex. These nutrients may act synergistically with each other and the rest of the nutrients in your supplemented Menus (that is to say, act together so that the total effectiveness is greater than the sum of the individual effectiveness of each cancer-preventive nutrient) to help counter the normal levels of carcinogens now inextricably woven into our lives.

But if you're exposed to higher-than-normal levels of carcinogens—if, for example, you're under severe stress, or you work in a plant that manufactures carcinogens or uses them as raw materials, or you smoke or spend a good part of the day with people who do, or you're on the Pill or on some therapeutic drugs, or if you're a sun-worshipper—then your supplemented Eat for Beautiful Skin Menus are likely to require augmentation with cancer-preventive nutrients. Whether that supplementation is necessary, and what quantities of nutrients are required if it is, is a matter that must be decided by your doctor.

Here's our personal nutritional formula to help prevent skin cancer (and other forms of cancer) when exposed to higher-than-normal levels of carcinogens:

> Vitamin A: 6,000 IU's
> Vitamin B-complex: one "100" product
> Vitamin C: 1,000 mg.
> Vitamin E: 400 IU's
> Selenium: 50 mcg.
> Zinc: 15 mg.

We take them as additional daily supplements to our supplemented Eat for Beautiful Skin Menus. We also enrich our menus with foods containing high quantities of the nutrients in the formula, making our selections from the charts in the Appendix, The 20 Best Sources of Selected Essential Nutrients. We substitute each food we select for a food in a matching Food Group in our Menus. As we pointed out in the preceding chapter, two members of the anti-oxidant team, nucleic acids and cysteine, need not be augmented because they're present in sufficient quantities in our Menus.

One final word of cancer-prevention advice: Do not go on any nutritional cancer preventive program, especially a program requiring supplementation, without the consent and supervision of your doctor.

Helping curb cancer. A pioneer in molecular biology, genetic structure, the immune system, the chemistry of the blood, and the chemistry of the mind; the creator of orthomolecular medicine—the bettering of human health through the right nutrients in the right amounts; recipient of two Nobel Prizes and 50-or-so honorary degrees; and author of more than 500 scientific papers, Dr. Linus Pauling is no David fighting the Goliath of the traditional medical cancer establishment. He's a colossus in his own right. This, in brief, is the story of his work in cancer.

By as early as 1954, many cancer investigators had understood that the deadliness of cancer lay not in the rapid and limitless proliferation of the cells (later to be the target of chemotherapy), but in the power of the cells to invade—penetrate, arrogate, destroy—healthy cells, tissues and organs. A little more than a decade later, a Scottish investigator, Dr. Ewan Cameron, discovered how cancer cells make that penetration. There's a "cement" between cells, collagen, that holds the cells together and surrounds each with a fortress-type wall. Cancer cells, jetting out an enzyme hyaluronidase, dissolves these walls and crashes through the debris into the healthy cells.

To Dr. Pauling, Dr. Cameron's description of the dissolution of the collagen walls was nothing new. It had been reported in scientific papers for more than a century. But not in connection with cancer. The liquefaction of collagen with its dread ultimate consequence—the body literally falling apart as the glue that held it together melts away—is the dominant symptom of scurvy. And scurvy is a disease caused by the deficiency of vitamin C.

Could vitamin C, then, control the invasiveness of cancer? The scientific literature, packed with correlations between vitamin C deficiency and cancer, encouraged Dr. Pauling. Perhaps, vitamin C, taken in adequate amounts could be the antihyaluronidase weapon that could stop the expansionist ravages of the cancer cells. When an enthusiastic Dr. Pauling proposed a test to Dr. Cameron, who had been looking for such an anticancer weapon, the Scottish investigator eagerly agreed.

In 1971, in the Vale of Levin Hospital, Loch Lomonside, Scotland, Cameron began daily administrations of 10,000 milligrams of vitamin C, as sodium ascorbate, to one hundred terminally ill cancer patients (called by Scottish doctors "the untreatables"—that is to say, patients for whom there was no treatment). The test lasted one year. The early results—a matter of days in some cases—were: a return of appetite, an increase in energy, and, most encouraging, so great a reduction in pain level that many patients no longer needed relief from narcotics. At years' end, patients who were expected to live only up to fifty days at the beginning of the test were still alive, and what's more, in vastly improved health, many showing no signs of malignancy. The test, it seemed, had proved more than what Drs. Pauling and Cameron had set out to prove. Not only could vitamin C counteract hyaluronidase and stop the spread of cancer cells, but it could also eradicate them.

Further work by Drs. Pauling and Cameron, as well as by independent Scandinavian investigators, demonstrated that vitamin C could increase the life-spans of terminal cancer patients by eight to eleven years. (These are unquestionably cures, in accordance with the American medical profession's definition of a cancer cure as any remedy that prolongs a patient's life by five years.) The ef-

fectiveness of vitamin C in cancer treatment is further corroborated, Dr. Pauling says, by the work of Dr. Fukimi Morishige in Ja-
pan who "like myself and Dr. Cameron believes so strongly in the
efficacy of vitamin C that he gives it to *all* of his patients." Dr. Pauling adds, "In China, [cancer] patients have been successfully
treated with vitamin C after physicians there had heard me lec-
ture [in 1981]."

But in one much-ballyhooed test conducted by the famed Mayo
Clinic in Rochester, Minnesota, the Pauling-Cameron vitamin theory was an utter failure. The test, though, was conducted on patients who had previously received extensive radiation therapy
and/or chemotherapy, treatments which, Drs. Pauling and Cameron had previously pointed out, would negate the effect of vitamin-C therapy. But in a Mayo Clinic re-test on patients who had
not undergone either of the objectionable therapies, vitamin-C
therapy failed again. Why the results in the two countries differ so
drastically is a mystery. One hypothetical solution: A high-nutrient-content diet in the Scottish hospital may have enhanced the
effects of vitamin C, while a low-nutrient-content diet in the American hospital may have inhibited it.

Currently Dr. Pauling heads the Linus Pauling Institute of Science and Medicine at Palo Alto, California. Although his ongoing research in cancer there is now partially funded, after many
years of rejections, by the National Cancer Institute, the Pauling-
Cameron vitamin C therapy is not standard medical practice.
Should a doctor treat a cancer patient with it exclusively (and it's
not effective any other way), and should the patient be harmed by
the treatment, the doctor may be liable for medical malpractice.

Another approach to the nutritional treatment of cancer has
been proposed by Dr. Virginia Livingston-Wheeler. She contends
that retinoids, close chemical relatives of vitamin A, not only are
anti-oxidants and help strengthen the immune system, but also
inhibit the action of a cancer-associated substance in the body
that may in part be responsible for the spread of cancer cells. She
includes retinoids, derived from fresh fruits and vegetables, as the
essential components of a nutritional program to combat cancer
by enhancing the body's immune system. Some beneficial effects
of retinoids in the treatment of some skin cancers have been reported in *The New England Journal of Medicine.* Dr. Livingston-
Wheeler has claimed "a remarkable rate of remission in cancer
patients" over the last fifteen years at her Livingston-Wheeler Med-

ical Clinic in San Diego, but her work has not been confirmed by independent studies.

As of now, there is no method of curbing cancer nutritionally that is accepted by conventional medicine (although some doctors are experimenting with vitamins as an adjunct to standard cancer therapy). But no tests have yet been conducted using a high-nutrient-content diet completely supplemented and augmented with massive doses of anti-oxidant and immune-system-boosting nutrients. When those tests are conducted, a new era in cancer therapy may be born, or the current era based on the hope that cancer may be curbed by nutritional therapy may come to an end.

11 Helping Keep Your Skin Beautiful Despite Stress, Smoking and the Pill

Run over in your mind the triggers that set off or exacerbate the skin conditions we've discussed in this book—from preclinical unattractiveness to acne, eczema, psoriasis, cancer, herpes and premature aging—and you'll find that stress is associated with all of them, and smoking and the Pill with unattractiveness and some of the serious disorders.

R_x advice for beautiful skin: Avoid stress. Quit smoking. Switch to an alternative contraceptive.

That's the best of advice; and in the best of all possible worlds it would be followed. But this isn't that world. In the U.S.A. of the eighties, stress comes with the territory; more than twenty million Americans refuse to believe smoking is a matter of life and breath; and two out of every five women between the ages of fifteen and forty-four regularly rely on the Pill. There's no extricating stress, smoking and the Pill from the American way of life.

And, strangely and sadly, it's questionable whether Americans truly *want* to extricate them. It's likely that we accept stress because we know there's a price to pay for the cornucopia of good-things-in-life that our society advertises, and stress is part of that price. We may smoke, not just because some of us have come a long way, baby, and others are riding the range in Marlboro Country, but because, mainly, tobacco soothes ruffled emotions, calms, comforts, and screens out distractions that threaten our capacity to work, and to work out our lives, efficiently. And chances are that women have an enduring love affair with the Pill because they know that, except for coitus interruptus practiced by a skillful and unselfish lover, no other contraceptive method can come close to offering a success rate of up to 99.5 percent.

What's the next best thing, then, for those of you who are unwilling or unable to free yourselves from stress, smoking and the Pill—any one of them or any combination? Some protection. Not complete, not perfect, not certain. But protection that gives you a reasonable chance to cut down overall adverse effects; and a realistic chance to help keep your skin beautiful. It's a chance that comes to you, as does every benefit in this book, from sound nutrition.

Helping keep your skin beautiful despite stress

Although psychosomatic medicine—the study of emotionally related physical illnesses—is nearly a century old, some conventional doctors are still uncomfortable with the stress-skin connection.

"Patients with acne or psoriasis ... will tell you they're doing well just prior to an examination or a job or a date," says Dr. Roland S. Medansky, a dermatologist who has researched the interplay between stress and skin disorders, "and all of a sudden they get worse. [But] can you prove this? Probably not."

Is the stress-skin connection real? Or is it a fantasy created by the patients for some reason of their own? Dr. Dorinda Shelley, a dermatologist with several scientific papers on stress and skin to her credit, supports the fantasy explanation, and thinks she knows the why of it. Patients desire to transform their repellent skin diseases into "a socially acceptable thing," she says. "They can have these awful [sores] on their skins and they'll say, 'It's due to my nerves.' ... Whereas, if they say they have something like psoriasis, it's ... different"—outside the pale of social acceptability.

But perhaps the real reason some conventional practitioners reject the stress-skin connection is that of all the interrelations between the emotions and the body—between the *psyche* and the *soma*—the one between stress and skin is the least understood by the medical profession. Nowhere in conventional medicine's archives is there a plan—a medical roadmap—tracing the physiological route from "an examination or a job or a date" to the painful, itch-maddening eye-sores of skin disorders, or to just common, everyday bad skin.

Yet there's not a medical encyclopedia or dermatological text that does not associate stress—"nerves"—with the onset and magnification of skin ailments. "The skin," says science writer Deborah Blumenthal, summing up the medical reportage on the subject, "can be a sensitive barometer of life's stresses. As one's mental state changes, so does the body, and particularly its most public aspect, the skin."

But *is* stress the cause? Or is it, as Dr. Shelley contends, the cover-up?

Nutritional scientists believe it's the cause; and in answer to Dr. Medansky's "Can you prove this?" they answer, "Yes. To a high degree of probability." They have, on their medical roadmaps, traced the routes from the feeling of stress to its depiction on the skin. Here, in broad outline, are those routes:

When you feel stress, the body responds with a burst of stress hormones to help you cope: to fight or flee, as dictated by genes as old as the fragile men-things that hunted the massive beasts of the Serengeti Plain tens of millions of years ago. With your survival at stake, the stress hormones demand, and receive, first priority for the raw materials of their manufacture. From the body's nutrient pool, and from the supply of ingested nutrients, what the stress-hormone factories need, they get. The other parts of the body are supplied in accordance with a hierarchy of priorities, and close to the bottom of that hierarchy is the skin.

Three things then can happen, separately or together.

One: The skin is deprived of nutrients; and the machinery for reproduction, growth and maintenance, dependent on a full supply of nutrients, falters into pathological errors.

Two: The anti-oxidant defense is weakened, and the rampaging oxidants (and their equally vicious immediate by-products, free radicals and superoxides) savage the cells' structure, invade the DNA, and cross-link the supple strands of collagen into the inflexible rods of old age.

And three: The stress hormones, created millenia ago to be dissipated by the biochemistry of fighting or fleeing, pile up in our sedentary bodies and degenerate into, and create, oxidants in massive numbers.

Replay in your mind the birth of the skin disorders in this book, superimpose on them one or more of the triple routes from stress to symptoms, and see how neatly they fit. They fit, too, for other skin disorders. Hives (urticaria)—a disease marked by sudden waterly swellings (wheals or welts) accompanied by pain and itching—may be the result of vitamin deprivation, notably of the B complex. Shingles (herpes zoster)—that herpes-virus disease related to chicken pox, characterized by a sudden outbreak of small blisters in a line around a side of the body, usually the torso—is possibly initiated by the deprivation of antioxidant defense nutrients, and the consequent destruction by oxidants of herpes virus-inhibiting amino acids. Lupus (systemic lupus erythematosus)—

the immune-system-breakdown disease manifested by a butterfly-shaped rash particularly on the cheeks and the bridge of the nose together with fever, anemia, arthritic pains and inflammation of the lungs—is likely to be the end-product of a massive oxidant attack on a nutrient-weakened immune system unsupported by a strong anti-oxidant team.

In the body's biochemistry, the stress-skin connection has every appearance of being real.

The treatment of stress-induced skin disorders, then, can be approached by living in a stress-free world (fine, if you can buy a one-way ticket to Shangri-La). Or by two in-this-world treatments: reducing or obliterating the feeling of stress, or the biochemical results of stress. Dermatologists who accept the stress-skin connection pragmatically ("Even if it's just in the patient's mind, let's get rid of it") prefer the first of the two therapies; nutritional scientists, the second.

To reduce or obliterate *the feeling of stress*—that is, the emotional effects of a stress situation—conventional dermatologists may include relaxation techniques in their courses of skin-disorder treatments: biofeedback, exercise, meditation, psychological counseling, even hobbies. Prescribed as well are tranquilizing drugs like valium and librium (together with their quotas of adverse side effects including possible addiction); but in tests conducted by Dr. Mendansky on eczema sufferers, no positive effects were found due to these drugs. (Possibly, because the drugs' calmative effects were offset by their nutrient-depleting and oxidant-producing effects.)

To reduce or obliterate *the biochemical results of stress*, nutritional scientists recommend that the nutrient pool, particularly the anti-oxidant defense, be built up to maximum strength. In everyday stress situations it *is* by your supplemented Eat for Beautiful Skin Menus. But nutrient augmentation of those Menus are needed when you're subjected to intense or chronic stress, such as job loss, death in the family, getting married, splitting up, being audited by the IRS, working at a job you don't like, taking examinations, experiencing sexual inadequacies, being arrested, participating in a law suit, contracting a venereal or other major disease, undergoing surgery, losing heavily in the stock market, going bankrupt, going on strike, being promoted or winning the sweepstakes.

Here's a nutrient anti-stress formula that we use, in conjunction with our supplemented Eat for Beautiful Skin Menus, when we're subjected to intense or chronic stress. Consult with your doctor about your need for such a formula and, should you need one, about what formula ingredients in what amounts are right for you.

> Vitamin A: 6,000 IU's
> Vitamin B-complex: one "100" product
> Vitamin B$_5$: 50 mg.
> Vitamin C: 1,000 mg.
> Vitamin E: 400 IU's
> Selenium: 50 mcg.
> Zinc: 15 mg.

Vitamin B$_5$ has been underscored because of its alleged qualities as an "anti-stress" vitamin. What that probably means is that under intense stress, for reasons not yet understood, the skin loses more of this vitamin than it does of others; hence, significant augmentation is necessary to undo the effects of stress. When there's a marked loss of vitamin B$_5$, fats and oils cannot be manufactured by the body in sufficient quantity, resulting in dry skin—a condition associated with intense stress.

We take the nutrients of the antistress formula as supplements, and we enrich our Eat for Beautiful Skin Menus with foods high in these nutrients. We choose these foods from the charts in the Appendix, The 20 Best Sources of Selected Essential Nutrients, and substitute each food for a food in a matching Food Group in the Menus.

Helping keep your skin beautiful despite smoking

Dr. C. Everett Koop, the Surgeon General of the United States, has characterized smoking as "the chief avoidable cause of death in our society and the most important public issue of our time. . . . We can say . . . today, with greater certainty than ever, that cigarettes are the most important individual health risk in this country, responsible for more premature death and disability than any other known agent."

In October 1984, the President of the United States, Ronald Reagan, signed legislation passed by the Congress requiring four different warnings from the Surgeon General to appear "conspicuously and prominently" in cigarette packages and advertising. The federal legislation mandates that the warnings be printed on a rotating basis, one every three months. They are:

SURGEON GENERAL'S WARNING: Smoking Causes Lung Cancer, Heart Disease, Emphysema, and May Complicate Pregnancy.

SURGEON GENERAL'S WARNING: Quitting Smoking Now Greatly Reduces Serious Risks to Your Health.

SURGEON GENERAL'S WARNING: Smoking by Pregnant Women May Result in Fetal Injury, Premature Birth, and Low Birth Weight.

SURGEON GENERAL'S WARNING: Cigarette Smoke Contains Carbon Monoxide.

Although there's no specific mention of the pernicious harm smoking does to the skin, this is the strongest antismoking action yet from the U.S. Government. It fortifies the efforts of such national organizations as the American Lung Association and ASH (Action on Smoking and Health) and of numerous statewide and local groups, to alert Americans to the dangers of smoking. Warned, each American then has the right under the laws of the land to slow-poison himself with cigarette smoke. Or not. (And the good news is that between 1981 and 1984, 20 percent more Americans than in the previous three years were deciding "not," according to statistics issued by the American Cancer Society.)

But when smokers exercise their right to flout the danger to themselves, they pass on the danger to nonsmokers who, for the most part, have no right to stop them. A study published in 1984 in *The New England Journal of Medicine* showed that a nonsmoking spouse inhaled, via smoke-polluted air, the equivalent of three cigarettes for every two packs consumed by the marital partner. If the predictions from a previous study were to hold true, then that spouse would die four years before the life-expectancy-chart age, have four times the anticipated risk of lung cancer, and live with the high probability of coming down with bronchitis and emphysema. Nonsmokers who work with smokers are often afflicted with damaged lungs; and children of parents who smoke are more likely to contract asthma, other respiratory disorders and ear infections than children in smoke-free households.

The point is: Even if you don't smoke, you may have to protect yourself from smoke. And your children, too.

The high risks to your skin from smoking come from the hazardous chemicals swirling in the tobacco fumes. The most dangerous of them are: the tars (polynuclear aromatic hydrocarbons); acetaldehyde (a chemical relative of formaldehyde, an ingredient of embalming fluid); heavy metals, such as lead and arsenic; radioactive polonium and radon particles ("radon daughters"); nicotine, which the body converts to carcinogenic nitrosamines; and nitrogen oxides and carbon monoxide.

Lead and arsenic are age-old ingredients of the poisoner's pharmacy; and carbon monoxide is the odorless, colorless, tasteless killer gas of automotive exhaust. The other ingredients, which affect the skin more perceptibly, initiate biochemical processes in the body that ultimately result in massive production of destructive oxidants. At the bottom of their scale of destructiveness is plain, everyday unattractive skin (look at another woman's skin, and eight times out of ten you can tell whether she smokes or whether she doesn't). Considerably higher on the scale is "smokers' skin," cross-linked, and, consequently, wrinkled, dry, inelastic, tough, aged, like a rubber windshield wiper or a garden hose ready for the junk heap. At the top of the scale: cancer.

There is no conventional medical approach to undoing the evils of smoking (not just cigarettes, but cigars, pipes, and the tobacco weed in any combustible form), but nutritional scientists offer several practical strategies, supported by convincing laboratory research.

One such strategy is based on decreasing the absorption of the poisons lead and arsenic. A combination of vitamins C and E; minerals copper, magnesium, iron, calcium and phosphorus; and the fiber, pectin (found in apples and other fruits) does it for lead. Vitamin C does it to some extent for arsenic. For the poisonous gas carbon monoxide, there's no antidote (hence the Surgeon General's specific warning against it). But carbon monoxide acts by preventing up to one out of five red blood cells in smokers' blood from carrying oxygen; and vitamin E may stimulate the oxygen-carrying capacity of the remaining red blood cells.

Another strategy aims to block the conversion of tobacco-smoke chemicals into carcinogens or oxidants. Vitamin C stands effectively in the way of nicotine becoming carcinogenic nitrosoamines. Acetaldehyde, particularly potent in forming cross-linkage oxidants, is neutralized by a nutrient team composed of vitamins B_1 and C and the amino acid cysteine. The radioactive heavy metals polonium and radon are kept in solution by vitamin C so they can be flushed out in the urine.

A final strategy targets the oxidants as they're produced. The antioxidant defense team, with which you've become familiar, are the destroyers.

All three strategies are linked together in this *nutrient smoking-protection formula*.

Nutrient	For smokers	For nonsmokers who live or work with smokers
Vitamin A	6,000 IU's	450 IU's
Vitamin B$_5$	50 mgs	10 mg.
Vitamin B$_6$	75 mgs	10 mg.
Vitamin C	1,000 mgs	500 mg.
Vitamin E	400 mgs	150 mg.
Selenium	50 mcgs	20 mcg.
Zinc	15 mgs	10 mg.
Copper	2 mgs	200 mcg.
Magnesium	1,000 mgs	75mg.
Iron	30 mgs	5 mg.
Calcium	1,200 mgs	75 mg.
Phosphorus	1,000 mgs	75 mg.

These nutrients should augment your supplemented Eat for Beautiful Skin Menus, subject to the approval and supervision of, and possible modification by, your doctor. At the same time, enrich your menus with foods high in the nutrients of the formula. Make your choices from the charts in the Appendix of The Twenty Best Sources of Selected Essential Nutrients. Substitute each choice for a food in a matching Food Group in your Menus.

Helping keep your skin beautiful despite the Pill

"Discontinue at once and call your doctor," warns Michele Paul, R.N., author of the authoritative *The Women's Pharmacy*, "if you experience any of the following symptoms: abdominal pains, blurred vision or loss of vision, chest pains, dizziness, flashing lights, numbness in arms or legs, severe leg pains, shortness of breath. These symptoms may indicate a blood clot or other serious condition." The other severe conditions to which she refers include heart attack, high blood pressure, headaches, depression, gall-bladder disorders, jaundice (a liver disorder), benign tumors, atherosclerosis, increased susceptibility to infections of the vagina, and cancer.

Michele Paul is writing about the Pill.

In the same major-health-hazard class as stress and smoking, the Pill, like the other two, leaves its marks on the public monitor of our health, the skin. Again from Paul: "The Pill ... causes or worsens acne, skin rashes, brown blotches on the skin ... and increases oiliness." It's also associated with melanomas of the benign and the malignant kind. (In fairness, it should be pointed out that some dermatologists prescribe the Pill for the treatment of acne. But we can find no supportive scientific test studies.)

The explanation of the Pill's baleful effects on the skin lies in the way it works:

Synthetic female hormones, chemicals that mimic estrogen and progesterone, kept daily at constant levels in the body, suppress the release of two other hormones, LH and FSH, responsible for the maturation of the egg in the ovary. Since the egg cannot mature, it cannot be released, and the sperm has nothing with which to mate. From the viewpoint of contraception: virtually perfect.

But from the viewpoint of the overall metabolism of the body: far from perfect. To maintain the constant level of female hormones day in and day out, the body must draw heavily on nutrients available from all parts of the body. The skin suffers the loss of some nutrients needed for cell reproduction, growth and maintenance; and some of the members of the antioxidant team are weakened to less-than-effective strength. The stage is set for the failure of the skin's health.

But it may be avoided by simply restoring the lost nutrients. You may do it with the following suggested formula based on studies of Pill-induced nutrient depletions. The formula should be used in conjunction with your supplemented Eat for Beautiful Skin Menus. Also enrich your Menus with choices from The 20 Best Sources of Selected Essential Nutrients in the Appendix. Remember that your nutrient requirements are different from any other woman's; so consult your doctor about your personal nutrient needs before you make any change in your diet.

Here is a nutrient formula to help protect against the Pill:

Vitamin B_1: 50 mg.
Vitamin B_2: 50 mg.
Vitamin B_6: 50 mg.
Vitamin B_{12}: 100 mcg.

Folic acid: 30 mg.
Vitamin C: 1,000 mg.
Vitamin E: 400 mg.
Zinc: 15 mgs.
Chromium: 500 mcg.

Chromium, a metal, is included in the formula, because it's necessary for maintaining a steady level of blood sugar (glucose tolerance), any deviation from which may in some cases result in poor skin.

Warning: The Pill decreases retinoid levels (another cause of poor skin) but increases vitamin-A levels, which theoretically should improve the health of the skin. That it doesn't may be attributed to the overwhelming antagonistic effects of other nutrient deprivations. At all events, with vitamin-A levels raised, it would be unwise to supplement your diet with that vitamin when you're on the Pill.

12 *Helping Keep Your Skin Beautiful Despite Sun and Surf*

"Bring back the parasol," exhort science writers Claudia Wallis and Mary Carpenter. "The Victorian ideal of delicate camelia-white skin has long been supplanted by the bronzed-[goddess] look. But the trend has taken a mortal toll. . . . The damage caused by [the sun's] rays range from ordinary sunburn to the wrinkles and liver spots [age spots] caused by years of sunbathing, to the precancerous dark patches known as actinic keratosis and finally, cancer." The surf adds an ironic insult of its own: Symbol of the ultimate wetness, it dries out your skin. And sun and surf together play the cruelest trick: To those of us who rush to the beaches of summer in quest of youthful skin, what happens, according to Temple University (Philadelphia) dermatologist Fred Urbach, is, "First you look old."

Sunlight, as all of us know who have ever directed its rays through a prism, is actually a rainbow of colors—violet, indigo, blue, green, yellow, orange and red in that order. Beyond one end of this spectrum are the invisible infrared rays; beyond the other, also out of the range of our eyesight, the ultraviolet and X rays. Infrared rays, big and lazy, warm the surface of the skin, but can't penetrate, don't burn. Ultraviolet rays and X rays, small and swift, can knife through the layers of the skin, burn, damage and destroy.

Fortunately, the ozone layer far above the highest cloudbanks is a giant radiation filter, holding back the sun's X rays and the most dangerous of its ultraviolet rays. The world's cloud cover absorbs about 20 percent of the ultraviolet rays that get through, and the rest pelts the earth, the beaches and the skins of sun-worshippers. Even if you're protected by a beach umbrella, richocheting rays, although reduced in strength by 75 percent, can target-in on you.

When they hit, in full or diluted strength, the ultraviolet rays rip through the skin's outer coat and scorch the cells near the surface, the basal cells. These, in a rapid emergency defense reaction, fill with cooling fluids. They swell. Blood, rushed to the site of the injury with restorative oxygen, nutrients and the body's own medicines, reddens the damaged region. The nerves in the skin scream with pain for more help. You're sunburned.

Continue exposure, and your body takes its last ditch defensive action. Melanin, the tan pigment that colors our skin, is shocked into overproduction, and rushed to the skin's surface where it spreads into a bronze barrier against the sun, turning away the insidious ultraviolet rays. The bronzed glamour of suntanned skin is the body's natural sunscreen.

Here's an itemized bill of the price we may pay for that glamour:

• *The sufferings of sunburn*, which range in intensity from redness, itching and mild pain to angry redness, blisters, severe pain, fever, headache, nausea and vomiting, followed in about a week by extensive peeling.

• *Premature aging*. The dry, wrinkled, inelastic skin of old age grows on us about 20 percent faster than on people who stay out of the sun. For every five days of our ardent sunbathing life our skin ages about six days. By our early thirties, the sun-splendid skin of our youth is in its late thirties; by our forties, it's in its fifties. In chronological old age, the skin may resemble a mummy's. Sunlight also hastens the growth and proliferation of age spots.

• *Keratosis* is at its least offensive when it appears in dark patches, at its worst when it erupts in hard, dark, horny growths. As keratosis lesions age, they tend to become malignant. "If we all live long enough," predicts Dr. Urbach, referring to the recent generations of sunbathers, "we would all get cancer."

• *Cancer*. The sun is responsible for four hundred thousand basal-cell carcinomas a year, sometimes directly, sometimes via the keratosis route. (The good news is, though: The cure rate is almost perfect.) But sun-induced malignant melanomas, which are virtually incurable, strike about fifteen thousand Americans yearly and kill about half of them. Of the two types of ultraviolet rays, shorter-wavelength UVB is the more carcinogenic; but longer wavelength UVA (you've already met it in the PUVA treatment of psoriasis) can also produce cancers.

• *Flare-ups of herpes, acne, psoriasis and other skin disorders*.

By contrast, the damage done directly by the surf is moderate: dryness. But indirectly it's flagrant: Sunlight reflected from water is many times as destructive as straight-on sunlight. (So is sunlight reflected from sandy beaches.)

Also having a multiplying effect on the damage potential of sunlight are stress, smoking and the Pill. Add these medicines, too: drugs containing antihistamines to treat cold, flu, sinus conditions and allergies; drugs, containing barbiturates and phenothiazines, for treatment of psychological disorders; antibiotics, including democycline, erythromycin and tetracycline; diuretics and anti-high blood pressure drugs containing thiazide; drugs to treat pain including aspirin and other salicylates; sulfonurea oral diabetes drugs; drugs, containing quinidine, to treat irregular heart rhythms; and drugs, containing quinine, to treat leg cramps and other leg disorders.

External protection against sun and surf

Sun-screen preparations are concocted to screen out some of the sun's harmful ultraviolet rays, UVA as well as UVB. Labels bear this rating: SPF followed by a number. SPF stands for Sun Protection Factor. The number indicates how much longer it will take to sunburn with a sunscreen preparation than *au naturel*. For example, SPF 2 indicates that it will take twice as long to sunburn with Tropical Blend Tequila Sunrise than with no protection; SPF 15, fifteen times longer with Sea & Ski Block Out.

The FDA divides sunbathers into four types according to the sunburn/tanning response of their skins to sunlight, and recommends SPF's for each type:

• For type I, skin that always burns and never tans (fair skin), SPF's of 9 to 15, with 15 preferred.

• For type II, skin that sometimes burns and never tans, SPF's of 6 to 8.

• For type III, skin that sometimes burns and tans well, SPF's of 4 to 8.

• For Type IV, for skin that never burns and tans beautifully (olive-toned skin), SPF's of 2 to 4.

Sun-screen products rated SPF 15 usually contain PABA (para-amino benzoic acid). It's a vitamin of the B complex that, besides having important skin-related functions inside the body, is so constructed that it can bounce back both UVA and UVB rays. As long ago as 1968, in a study comparing twenty-four commercial sunscreen preparations, those containing PABA proved the most effective. Available today in numerous commercial sun-screen preparations, PABA, though, has its drawbacks: It can irritate skin; stain fabrics; and when used in conjunction with any of the sunlight-damage-multiplying drugs described previously in this chapter, can lose much of its protective capability. There are nonstaining varieties of PABA-containing sun screens on drugstore shelves, but they're not as effective as those that can stain.

Some sun-screen preparations, with or without PABA, are water-proof (stay on in the surf for at least eighty minutes); non-pore-blocking (avoiding mechanically produced skin disorders); oil-free (for when your skin is oily enough); fragrance-free (for that fresh, clean, natural scent); non-irritating (gentled down for use on the more sensitive parts of the body including the face); and moisturizing.

Subjected regularly to the depradations of sun and surf, sun-bathers need moisturizers off-beach as well as on. Moisturizers, contrary to popular belief, do not assure the dewy freshness of skin by working oil into the cells; but, rather, by forming a thin layer of oil, or other protectant, on the skin to prevent evaporation of water already there. That's why moisturizers work better when applied to damp skin—skin fresh from the surf, bath or shower; and that's why moisturizing creams, which contain more oil than lotions, work better than lotions.

Best moisturizers, according to "well-designed studies" reported by science writer Jane E. Brody, are lanolin, a purified wool fat mixed with water to give it a thick oily consistency, and petroleum jelly, the major component of Vaseline and similar products. "Applied once a day for three weeks," Brody states, "these resisted dryness for up to three weeks after their use was discontinued." She also recommends baby oil (light mineral oil with a fragrance) as a superior moisturizer. Olive oil gets the hearty approval of nutritional scientist, Dr. Michael A. Weiner. "In Mediterranean countries," he writes, "olive oil has been rubbed on the skin to lubricate it and prevent loss of moisture since antiquity."

Another moisturizing technique is to attract moisture to the skin. There are chemicals called humectants that absorb water from the air, and consequently impart moisture to anything with which they're in contact. Glycerine is such a chemical; and glycerine preparations, applied to the skin, are successful moisturizers. Your skin has its own humectant. It's Na-PCA (the sodium salt of 2-pyrrolidone-5-carboxylic acid). "The ability of Na-PCA to pull water out of the air," writes Durk Pearson and Sandy Shaw, "is amazing. If you put out a small amount of dry Na-PCA in the Sahara, in a few hours it will become a puddle because of the water removed from the very dry air there." Pearson and Shaw contend that sun and surf lead to dry skin by leaching out the natural Na-PCA. They suggest that Na-PCA-containing cosmetics, on sale in some health-food stores, can restore this potent humectant to the skin.

But that a naturally occurring internal component of the skin can be utilized by the skin when applied externally has not received universal medical acceptance. Dr. Susan E. Mackel, professor of dermatology at the University of Virginia School of Medicine, voicing the opinion of most dermatologists, says, as reported by Jane E. Brody, that "there is no scientifically documented reason to invest in cosmetics that contain vitamins ... or other supposedly natural ingredients." Standard medical thinking holds that the skin cannot be fed from the outside.

Nutritional scientists believe that it can. "Some of the nutrients recommended as dietary supplements," writes Dr. Weiner, "are also beneficial when applied externally. Vitamin E oil and vitamins A and D ointments are among the best treatments for dry skin." But conventional dermatologists Drs. Arnold W. Klein and James H. Sternberg warn that vitamin-E skin preparations have no healing powers, and can induce skin rashes among people allergic to vitamin E.

Familiar face makeup, though, does get the nod of approval from some dermatologists as a barrier against sunlight during nonbeach exposure, particularly when the cosmetics have sunscreens and oil bases, which act as moisturizers. But cosmetics, which are not required to meet FDA requirements for safety and effectiveness prior to marketing, may not work for that purpose, and may carry the threat of itching, rashes, and other skin irritations.

Here are our assessments of skin preparations to fight sun and surf. Sun-screen creams and lotions, particularly those containing PABA, make good sense. The time-tested moisturizers we've mentioned—lanolin, olive oil, and so on—do the job. But the effectiveness of topical Na-PCA has yet to be proved beyond a reasonable doubt; and that of Vitamins A, E, and D moisturizers is questionable. Makeup is essentially for cosmetic purposes, and should not be solely relied upon for skin protection. All protectants against sun and surf may irritate the skin and/or provoke allergic reactions.

Internal protection against sun and surf

Conventional dermatologists concede that the action of the sun's ultraviolet rays suppresses the immune system, accounting for flare-ups of herpes-virus infections (herpes simplex I and II, and chicken pox among others) when the body is exposed to protracted sunlight. Dr. Margaret Kripke of the National Cancer Institute, moreover, sees in the immune system suppression a possible "aggravating factor in the development of skin cancer."

Nutritional scientists agree, but add that UVA and UVB rays also do considerable damage through the production of oxidants, including one of the most potent of that devasting group of chemicals, singlet oxygen. A pernicious carcinogen that targets-in on the DNA and RNA of cells, it also attacks fats and proteins, crosslinking them into lipofuscin, a yellow-brown waste material that emerges on the skin as age spots.

The suppression of the immune system and the expansion of the oxidant population is associated, as we've already seen, with nutrient deficiencies. The restoration of the body's nutrient pool to a level sufficient to provide maximum strength to the immune system and the antioxidant defense becomes the overriding strategy for helping protect the skin against the ravages of sun and surf. Here's how to execute that strategy:

A nutritional formula to help prevent mild adverse effects of sun and surf. Supplement your Eat for Beautiful Skin Menus with two—not one—multi-vitamin/mineral products daily, during the period when you're exposed to sun and surf. In addition, add 100 milligrams of potassium orotate (available in health-food and drug stores), which may help build significant quantities of Na-PCA, the skin's natural moisturizer. Potassium orotate is a derivative, of orotic acid, which has been called vitamin B_{13}. This formula, to be used only with the approval of your doctor (additional potassium may be undesirable), may help protect against intermittent mild exposure to sunlight. For protracted intense exposure, the formulas to help protect against premature skin aging (page 77) and skin cancer (page 88) may be more effective. Consult your doctor about your individual needs.

III

Cooking for Beautiful Skin

13 *Eat for Beautiful Skin Recipes*

If you're a woman whose life is filled with things-to-do (and what woman's life isn't?), you'll want recipes that are quick and easy. These are.

If you've often longed for healthful recipes that are homespun and as American as apples and pie, your days of longing are over.

If you're fed up with women's-mag recipes that sugar-and-cream you with extra pounds, and you're desperate for taste-as-goods with calorie-control, here they are.

If you shrink from the thought of preparing one meal for yourself and another meal for the rest of the family, and would give anything for healthful recipes that please all tastes, you've got them.

If you've daydreamed of a sleep-in nutritionist or, better, a computer that could print out maximum-nutrition recipes for you, here's the print-out.

If your three favorite qualities of a recipe are in ascending order: 1. Taste 2. Taste 3. Taste—you've got all three.

And . . .

If you want model recipes that are filled to the brim with good-for-the-skin foods, so you can model your own recipes on them, start modeling.

Fact is, you can come up with your own Eat for Beautiful Skin recipes, as the recipes in this chapter demonstrate, by making a few replacements (for the better) in your own recipes: vegetable oils for lard or hydrogenated fats, skim milk for cream, honey for white sugar, herbs and spices for excess salt, and most important good-for-your-skin foods for bad-for-your-skin foods (let Chapters 2 and 4 be your shopping Bible).

One last bonus: You don't have to go to health-food stores, exotic gourmet shops or send away to far-off places with strange-sounding names to get the ingredients for your recipes. Your neighborhood supermarket has them all. And the price, like the food, is right. So *Eat for Beautiful Skin* hassle-free, economically and deliciously.

Five Fish Dishes

BAKED LEMON HALIBUT

1	pound Halibut fillet	⅛	teaspoon salt, if desired
1	tablespoon butter or vegetable oil	Dash	pepper
4	teaspoons lemon juice	⅛	teaspoon rosemary
1	teaspoon grated lemon rind		

1. Preheat oven to 350 degrees F. (moderate).

2. Divide fish into 6 servings. Place in single layer in baking pan.

3. Mix fat, lemon juice, lemon rind, salt, pepper and rosemary. Pour over fish.

4. Bake for 25 minutes or until fish flakes easily when tested with a fork.

Serves 6, about 2 ounces each.
Calories per serving: 130.

BAKED STUFFED HADDOCK

1	pound haddock	4	teaspoons chopped parsley
2	teaspoons vegetable oil	¼	teaspoon sage
¼	cup chopped onion	¼	teaspoon salt, if desired
¼	cup chopped celery	⅛	teaspoon pepper
2	cups whole-wheat bread cubes, soft	1	tablespoon butter

1. Grease shallow baking pan with oil.
2. Heat oil in small frying pan. Add onion and celery.
3. Cover and cook, stirring occasionally, until vegetables are tender.
4. Stir in bread cubes, 3 teaspoons of the parsley, sage, salt and pepper.
5. Arrange half of fillets in the baking pan. Top with remaining fillets.
6. Cover and bake at 325 degrees F. (slow oven) for 15 minutes.
7. Mix butter with remaining parsley. Spoon over fish fillets. Continue baking, uncovered, until fish flakes easily when tested with a fork, about ten minutes.

Serves 4, about 3 ounces each.
Calories per serving: 69.

DEVILED SCROD PATTIES

1½	pounds scrod fillets		1	egg
1	cup boiling water		1	tablespoon prepared mustard
¼	teaspoon salt, if desired		1	tablespoon lemon juice
½	cup bread crumbs, soft		1	teaspoon Worcestershire sauce
2	tablespoons parsley, chopped		⅛	teaspoon pepper
½	cup Sour Creamy Dressing (page 138)			paprika to taste

1. Preheat oven to 400 degrees F. (hot)

2. Grease baking sheet.

3. Add fish to boiling, salted water. Cover and bring to a boil. Reduce heat and cook 4 minutes or until fish flakes easily. Drain and flake. Remove bones, if any.

4. Mix fish, bread crumbs and parsley.

5. Mix salad dressing, egg, mustard, lemon juice, Worcestershire sauce and pepper thoroughly. Stir into fish mixture. Mix well.

6. Form into 12 patties about 3 inches in diameter and ¾ inch thick, and lay on baking sheet.

7. Sprinkle with paprika.

8. Bake 15 to 20 minutes or until lightly browned.

Serves 6, two patties each.
Calories per serving: 235.

FISH CHOWDER

1	pound Haddock fillets without skin	2	tablespoons water
1½	cups ¼-inch diced potatoes	2	cups skim milk
2	tablespoons chopped onions	½	teaspoon salt, if desired
1	cup boiling water	Dash	pepper
2	tablespoons flour	1	tablespoon butter

1. Cut fish into 1-inch pieces

2. Add fish, potatoes and onion to boiling water. Cover and simmer until potatoes are just tender, about 10 minutes. Drain.

3. Mix flour with 2 tablespoons water until smooth. Stir into milk.

4. Add milk mixture, salt and pepper to fish mixture. Cook, stirring gently until thickened.

5. Stir in butter.

Serves 4, about 1 cup each.
Calories per serving: 205.

BAKED FLOUNDER FILLETS

1	*pound flounder fillet*	½	*teaspoon salt, if desired*
2	*teaspoons melted butter*	¼	*teaspoon paprika*
1	*tablespoon lemon juice*	1	*teaspoon chopped parsley*

1. Lightly grease a shallow baking pan.

2. Place fillets in a single layer, skin side down, in pan.

3. Mix butter, lemon juice, salt and paprika. Spoon over fillets.

4. Bake at 350 degrees F. (moderate oven) until fish flakes easily when tested with a fork, about 20 minutes.

5. Garnish each serving with parsley.

Serves 4, about 3 ounces each.
Calories per serving: 115.

Four Chicken Dishes and One Turkey Dish

LEMON BAKED CHICKEN

3	tablespoons lemon juice		¼	teaspoon salt, if desired
2	tablespoons vegetable oil		⅛	teaspoon paprika
1	tablespoon minced onion		4	chicken breast halves, without skin

1. Mix all ingredients except chicken.
2. Place chicken pieces in shallow baking pan.
3. Pour lemon mixture over chicken pieces.
4. Bake at 400 degrees F. (hot oven) until chicken is tender, about 1 hour. Baste chicken several times with liquid in pan during baking.

Serves 4, 1 chicken breast half each.
Calories per serving: 190.

CHICKEN CURRY

¼	cup onion, chopped	1	teaspoon curry powder
2	cups tart apple, unpared, chopped	1	cup skim milk
1	tablespoon vegetable oil	1½	cups cooked, diced chicken
2	tablespoons flour	¼	cup raisins
½	teaspoon salt, if desired	2	cups cooked brown rice, unsalted
⅛	teaspoon ground ginger		

1. Cook onion and apple in oil until tender.
2. Stir in flour, salt, ginger and curry powder.
3. Add milk slowly, stirring constantly. Cook until thickened.
4. Add chicken and raisins. Heat to serving temperature.
5. Serve over rice.

Serves 4, about ⅔ cup curry and ½ cup rice each.
Calories per serving: 290.

CHICKEN CROQUETTES

2	tablespoons chopped onions	1/8	teaspoon poultry seasoning
1/4	cup chopped celery	3/4	cup skim milk
2	tablespoons vegetable oil	2	cups finely minced chicken, cooked
1/3	cup flour	1	tablespoon butter
1/4	teaspoon salt, if desired	1/2	cup bread crumbs
1/8	teaspoon pepper	1	recipe mushroom sauce (see page 134)

1. Cook onion and celery in oil until onion is clear.
2. Stir in flour and seasonings.
3. Add milk slowly, stirring constantly. Cook until thickened.
4. Mix chicken with milk mixture.
5. Chill thoroughly.
6. Shape chilled chicken mixture into 8 croquettes.
7. Mix margarine with bread crumbs.
8. Roll croquettes in crumb mixture. Place on baking sheet.
9. Bake at 400 degrees F. (hot oven) until lightly browned, about 30 minutes.
10. Serve with mushroom sauce.

Serves 4, two croquettes each.
Calories per serving without sauce: 305.

CHICKEN SALAD

2	cups diced, cooked chicken		½	teaspoon salt, if desired
½	cup chopped celery		1	tablespoon lemon juice
⅔	cup diced tart apple, with skin			salad greens to taste (try to include sprouts and alfalfa)
½	cup grapes, seedless or seeded halves			
½	cup vegetable-oil dressing			

1. Tossing gently, mix chicken, celery, apple and grapes together.
2. Mix salad dressing, salt and lemon juice.
3. Gently stir salad dressing mixture into chicken mixture.
4. Chill well.
5. Serve on crisp salad greens.

Serves 4, about 1 cup each.
Calories per serving: 185.

TURKEY TETRAZZINI

1	can (2 ounces) mushroom stems and pieces	1½	cups cooked, diced turkey
2	tablespoons chopped green pepper	1	tablespoon pimiento, chopped
2	tablespoons vegetable oil	2	tablespoons sherry, if desired
3	tablespoons flour	2	cups cooked, thin spaghetti (about 4 ounces uncooked), unsalted
½	teaspoon salt, if desired	1	tablespoon Parmesan cheese, grated
Dash	pepper		
½	cup turkey or chicken broth		
1	can (13 fluid ounces) evaporated skim milk		

1. Grease 1½-quart casserole lightly with oil.

2. Cook mushrooms and green pepper in oil until green pepper is tender.

3. Stir in flour, salt, and pepper.

4. Mix broth with milk. Add slowly to flour mixture, stirring constantly. Cook until thickened.

5. Stir in turkey, pimiento and sherry.

6. Mix in spaghetti.

7. Pour into casserole. Sprinkle with cheese.

(continued)

8. Bake at 350 degrees F. (moderate oven) until bubbly throughout, about 30 minutes.

Serves 4, about 1 cup each.
Calories per serving: 385 with sherry; 375 without.

Four Meat Dishes and One Egg Dish

BAKED LOUISIANA PORK CHOPS

¼ cup chopped onion

¼ cup chopped green pepper

2 teaspoons vegetable or olive oil

1 8-ounce can tomatoes

¼ teaspoon salt, if desired

⅛ teaspoon pepper

4 loin pork chops (about 4 ounces)

1. Cook onion and green pepper in oil until onion is clear.

2. Break up large pieces of tomatoes.

3. Add tomatoes, salt and pepper to cooked onion and green pepper.

4. Cover and simmer 20 minutes to blend flavors.

5. Trim fat from chops.

6. Brown chops lightly on both sides in hot frying pan. Place in baking pan.

7. Pour sauce over chops.

8. Cover and bake at 350 degrees F. (moderate oven) until chops are tender, about 45 minutes.

Serves 4, 1 chop each.
Calories per serving: 155.

BEEF BURGUNDY

¾	pound beef round, well-trimmed, cut into 1-inch cubes	½	cup diced celery
		⅓	cup chopped onions
¼	teaspoon salt, if desired	1	cup sliced onions
⅛	teaspoon pepper	3	tablespoons whole-wheat flour
1	bay leaf	¼	cup water
⅛	thyme leaves	⅓	cup red burgundy wine, if desired
1½	cups water		
1½	cups diced potatoes		parsley, as garnish
1	cup sliced carrots		

1. Brown beef cubes in hot frying pan.

2. Add salt, pepper, bay leaf, thyme and 1½ cups water.

3. Simmer, covered, until beef is almost tender, about 1¾ hours.

4. Remove bay leaf.

5. Add potatoes, carrots, celery, onion and mushrooms. Simmer, covered, until vegetables are tender, about 20 minutes.

6. Mix flour with ¼ cup water until smooth. Add slowly to meat mixture, stirring gently. Cook until thickened.

7. Stir in wine.

8. Serve, garnished with parsley.

Serves 4, about 1 cup each.
Calories per serving: 225.

ITALIAN GROUND BEEF AND MACARONI

¾	pound ground beef, extra-lean	1	teaspoon dried oregano
½	cup chopped onion	1	teaspoon dried basil
¼	cup chopped green pepper	¼	teaspoon salt, if desired
¼	cup chopped celery	⅛	teaspoon black pepper
1	16-ounce can tomatoes	3	cups elbow macaroni (about 1 cup uncooked), unsalted
1	¾-ounce can tomato purée		

1. Cook beef, onion, green pepper and celery in large frying pan until beef is lightly browned and onion is clear. Drain.

2. Break up large pieces of tomato.

3. Add tomatoes, tomato purée and seasonings to beef mixture. Simmer 15 minutes to blend flavors.

4. Stir in macaroni. Heat to serving temperature.

Serves 4, about 1⅓ cups each.
Calories per serving: 330.

BROILED STEAK WITH CREOLE SAUCE

¼ cup chopped onion	¼ teaspoon salt, if desired
¼ cup chopped green pepper	⅛ teaspoon pepper
2 teaspoons olive oil	1 pound beef round steak, boneless
1 8-ounce can tomatoes	

1. Cook onion and green pepper in oil until onion is clear.

2. Break up large pieces of tomatoes.

3. Add tomatoes, salt and pepper to cooked onion and green pepper.

4. Cover and simmer 20 minutes to blend flavors.

5. Trim fat from steak.

6. Brown steak lightly on both sides in hot frying pan. Place in baking dish.

7. Pour sauce over steak.

8. Cover and bake at 350 degrees F. (moderate oven) until steak is tender, about 1½ hours.

Serves 4, about 2¼ ounces each.
Calories per serving: 190.

WESTERN OMELETTE

2	teaspoons very finely minced onion	1	teaspoon salt, if desired
		Dash	pepper
1	tablespoon very finely minced green pepper	½	cup cooked, chopped pork
1	teaspoon butter	2	tablespoons finely chopped pimiento
¼	cup skim milk		
4	eggs, slightly beaten	2	tablespoons chopped parsley

1. Cook onion and green pepper in covered nonstick frypan until tender.

2. Mix milk, eggs, salt and pepper. Beat until frothy.

3. Pour egg mixture into pan with onion and green pepper.

4. Cook, stirring occasionally, until eggs begin to set.

5. Stir in pork, pimiento and parsley.

6. Cook until eggs are set.

Serves 4, about ⅓ cup each.
Calories per serving: 130.

Seven Vegetable Dishes

CORN CHOWDER

1	12-ounce can vacuum-packed whole kernel corn	2	cups skim milk
1½	cups ¼-inch diced potatoes	½	teaspoon salt, if desired
		Dash	black pepper
2	tablespoons chopped onion	1	tablespoon butter
2	tablespoons corn liquid from can		

1. Drain corn. Set corn and liquid aside.

2. Add potatoes and onions to boiling water. Cover and simmer until potatoes are just tender, about 10 minutes.

3. Mix flour with 2 tablespoons corn liquid until smooth. Stir into milk.

4. Add milk mixture, corn, salt and pepper to potato-onion mixture. Cook, stirring gently until thickened.

5. Stir in butter.

Serves 4, about 1 cup each.
Calories per serving: 180.

RICE AND BEANS

½	cup chopped onion	2	cups cooked rice
½	cup chopped celery	1	tablespoon chopped parsley
1	clove garlic, minced		
2	tablespoons butter or vegetable oil	¼	teaspoon salt, if desired
1	16-ounce can kidney beans	⅛	teaspoon pepper

1. Cook onion, celery and garlic in butter or oil until tender.
2. Add remaining ingredients.
3. Simmer together for 5 minutes to blend flavors.

Serves 6, about ½ cup each.
Calories per serving: 165.

HEARTY BEAN STEW

1	cup dry navy (pea) beans or soybeans	1	bay leaf
4	cups boiling water	⅛	teaspoon pepper
½	cup sliced onion	1	cup sliced carrots
1	cup cooked, diced lean fresh ham	¼	cup diced celery
¼	teaspoon salt, if desired	2	teaspoons whole-wheat flour
		1	tablespoon water

1. Add beans to boiling water. Return to boil.

2. Boil 2 minutes. Remove from heat, cover and soak 1 hour.

3. Return to boiling. Add onion, ham and seasonings. Boil uncovered for 5 minutes, then cover and boil gently until beans are almost tender, about 1 hour.

4. Add carrots and celery. Cook until tender, about 20 minutes.

5. Remove bay leaf.

6. Mix flour with 1 tablespoon water until smooth. Add slowly to beans, stirring constantly. Cook until thickened.

Note: Ham may be omitted.
Serves 4, about 1 cup each.
Calories per serving: with ham, 265; without ham, 165.

SWEET POTATOES WITH PINEAPPLE

½   tablespoon butter or
    vegetable oil

¼   teaspoon ground
    cinnamon

2   cups cooked, sliced
    fresh sweet potatoes

⅛   teaspoon salt, if
    desired

1   8-ounce can crushed
    pineapple in natural
    juice

1. Heat oil in large frying pan. Add potato slices and pineapple. Sprinkle with cinnamon and salt.

2. Simmer, uncovered, until most of the juice has evaporated, about 10 to 15 minutes. Turn potato slices several times.

Serves 4, about ½ cup each.
Calories per serving: 135.

COTTAGE CHEESE BAKED POTATOES

2	8-ounce baked potatoes	¼	teaspoon salt, if desired
½	cup cottage cheese, dry-curd, low-fat	⅛	teaspoon pepper
			paprika to taste
¼	cup skimmed milk		

1. Wash potatoes well. Prick skins in several places. Bake at 425 degrees F. (hot oven) until tender, 50 to 60 minutes.

2. Remove from oven, cut in half. Scoop out inside of potatoes, leaving skins intact. Save skins. Mash potatoes thoroughly.

3. Add remaining ingredients except paprika. Beat until fluffy.

4. Put mashed-potato mixture into potato skins. Sprinkle paprika over the tops.

5. Bake at 425 degrees until heated through and tops are lightly browned, about 10 minutes.

Serves 4, half a potato each.
Calories per serving: 110.

PEAS VINAIGRETTE

1	16-ounce can peas	½	tablespoon honey
⅓	cup onion, sliced	¼	teaspoon dry mustard
¼	cup green pepper, chopped	⅛	teaspoon salt, if desired
2	tablespoons vinegar	Dash	pepper
2	tablespoons vegetable oil		

1. Heat peas to boiling. Drain.
2. Lightly mix peas, onion and green pepper.
3. Mix vinegar, oil, honey and seasonings thoroughly.
4. Stir into vegetable mixture.
5. Chill well, stirring occasionally.

Serves 4, about ½ cup each.
Calories per serving: 190.

MUSHROOM SAUCE

1	tablespoon vegetable oil	¾	cup skim milk
1½	tablespoons flour	1	2-ounce can mushrooms, sliced, drained
¼	teaspoon salt, if desired		

1. Heat oil. Stir in flour and salt.

2. Add milk slowly, stirring constantly. Cook until thickened.

3. Add mushrooms. Heat to serving temperature.

Serves 4, about ¼ cup each.
Calories per serving: 60.

Four Salad Dressings

SAVORY SALAD DRESSING

2	tablespoons corn starch	⅛	teaspoon paprika
¼	cup honey	1	cup skim milk
1	teaspoon salt, if desired	4	egg whites
		¼	cup vinegar
1	teaspoon dry mustard	1	tablespoon olive oil

1. Mix dry ingredients in saucepan. Stir in milk.
2. Cook over low heat, stirring constantly until thickened.
3. Beat egg whites until frothy.
4. Add some of hot mixture slowly to egg whites, stirring constantly.
5. Add egg white mixture slowly to remaining hot mixture, stirring constantly. Cook until thickened. Remove from heat.
6. Add vinegar and olive oil. Mix well.
7. Chill before serving. Store in refrigerator.

Makes about 1⅔ cups.
Calories per tablespoon: 20.

FRENCH-STYLE DRESSING

1½	tablespoons cornstarch	¼	cup dry mustard
2	tablespoons sugar	½	teaspoon paprika
1	cup water	⅛	teaspoon onion powder
¼	cup vinegar	Dash	garlic powder

1. Mix cornstarch and sugar in saucepan. Stir in water.
2. Cook over low heat, stirring constantly until thickened.
3. Cool slightly.
4. Add remaining ingredients. Mix thoroughly.
5. Chill.

Makes about 1 cup.
Calories per tablespoon: 10.

DILL-YOGURT DRESSING

1	8-ounce container plain low-fat yogurt	½	teaspoon dill weed, crushed
2	teaspoons onion, very finely chopped	¼	teaspoon dry mustard
1	teaspoon lemon juice	⅛	teaspoon garlic powder

1. Mix all ingredients thoroughly.

2. Chill until served.

Makes about 1 cup.
Calories per tablespoon: 10.

SOUR CREAMY DRESSING

½   cup dry-curd, low-fat
    cottage cheese

¼   cup buttermilk

1   tablespoon vegetable
    oil

1   teaspoon lemon
    juice

⅛   teaspoon salt, if
    desired

1. Put all ingredients into blender container. Cover.

2. Blend until smooth.

Makes about ⅔ cup.
Calories per tablespoon: 20.

Four Desserts and One Dessert Topping

PEACHY YOGURT PIE

For the pie shell:

1   cup whole-wheat flour

½   teaspoon salt, if desired

2   tablespoons water

¼   cup vegetable oil

For the filling:

1   16-ounce can sliced peaches in light syrup

1   envelope unflavored gelatin

⅓   cup frozen orange juice

¹⁄₁₆ teaspoon almond extract

¼   teaspoon vanilla extract

1   8-ounce container plain low-fat yogurt

To make the pie shell:

1. Mix flour and salt thoroughly.

2. Mix 3 tablespoons flour mixture with the water to make a paste.

3. Using a fork, lightly mix oil with remaining flour mixture until mixture is crumbly.

4. Stir flour paste into flour-oil mixture to form a ball.

5. Roll dough between two sheets of wax paper until the dough is at last an inch wider all around than the pie pan. Remove top paper.

6. Invert pastry paper-side-up over pie pan. Pull off remaining paper. Fit carefully into pie pan, lifting edges as necessary to

(continued)

eliminate air bubbles. Trim off irregular edges of dough, leaving about ½ inch beyond rim of pan. Fold dough under to edge of pan.

7. Flute edge of dough with fingers or press lightly to pan with tines of fork. Prick bottom and side well with fork.

8. Bake at 450 degrees F. (very hot oven) until lightly browned, about 11 minutes. Cool.

To make the filling:

1. Drain peaches. Save liquid. Coarsely chop peaches.

2. Mix gelatin with peach liquid.

3. Heat mixture, stirring constantly until gelatin is dissolved.

4. Stir in orange-juice concentrate and extracts.

5. Chill until mixture is consistency of egg whites. Whip until fluffy.

6. Fold in yogurt. Add peaches.

7. Add honey sweetener, if desired.

8. Pour into pie shell.

9. Chill until set.

Makes 9-inch pie, serves 8.
Calories per serving: 180.

GINGER WHEAT COOKIES

½	cup butter	1	teaspoon baking soda
½	cup honey	¼	teaspoon salt, if desired
2	eggs		
⅓	cup orange juice	¼	teaspoon ground cloves
2	cups whole-wheat flour	2	teaspoons ground ginger
½	cup wheat germ, unsweetened	½	cup chopped raisins

1. Preheat oven to 350 degrees F. (moderate).

2. Mix butter and honey.

3. Add eggs and orange juice. Beat vigorously.

4. Mix dry ingredients thoroughly.

5. Add dry ingredients and raisins to oil mixture. Mix well.

6. Drop dough by teaspoonfuls onto ungreased baking sheet, about 2 inches apart.

7. Bake until lightly browned and cookie feels firm to the touch, about 8 minutes.

8. Remove from baking sheet while still warm.

9. Cool on rack.

Makes about 60 cookies.
Calories per cookie: 55.

STEAMED CARROT PUDDING

½	cup whole-wheat flour	¼	teaspoon ground nutmeg
¼	teaspoon baking powder	1	egg
¼	teaspoon baking soda	1	tablespoon butter
⅓	cup honey	½	cup grated carrots
⅛	teaspoon salt, if desired	½	cup grated potatoes
½	teaspoon ground cinnamon	¼	cup grated lemon rind
		2	tablespoons grated walnuts

1. Grease a 2½ cup casserole or small pudding mold.
2. Mix together dry ingredients.
3. Beat egg and butter together. Stir in flour mixture. Mix well.
4. Add remaining ingredients. Mix well.
5. Pour mixture into casserole. Cover tightly with foil.
6. Place casserole on rack in deep pan. Add boiling water until it comes halfway up side of casserole. Casserole should not touch lid of pan.
7. Cover pan and simmer 2 hours.
8. Remove casserole from pan. Cool on rack until lukewarm.
9. Unmold pudding from casserole.
10. Serve warm or cool completely.

Note: To store, wrap in foil and place in refrigerator. For best quality use within 4 to 5 days.
Serves 8.
Carlories per serving: 105.

WHOLE WHEAT BISCUITS

1	cup whole-wheat flour	½	teaspoon salt, if desired
1	cup all-purpose flour	⅔	cup skim milk
2½	teaspoons baking powder	⅓	cup vegetable oil

1. Preheat oven to 450 degrees F. (very hot).
2. Mix dry ingredients thoroughly.
3. Mix milk and oil.
4. Make a depression in center of dry ingredients. Pour in liquid mixture all at once.
5. Stir with a fork until dough separates from side of bowl.
6. Knead dough gently on a lightly floured surface 18 times.
7. Roll to ½-inch thicknesses.
8. Cut with a 2-inch cookie cutter.
9. Place on ungreased baking sheet.
10. Bake until lightly browned, about 12 minutes.

Note: Serve plain or with low-calorie or nonsweetened jam or jelly.
Makes 12 biscuits.
Calories per biscuit: 120.

LOW-CALORIE WHIPPED TOPPING

1	teaspoon unflavored gelatin	½	cup skim milk
2	teaspoons water	½	teaspoon vanilla
¼	cup instant nonfat dry milk	1	tablespoon honey, if desired

1. Soften gelatin in water for 5 minutes.
2. Stir nonfat dry milk into skim milk in saucepan. Heat to simmering. Add softened gelatin. Stir until gelatin is dissolved.
3. Add vanilla and honey.
4. Chill until mixture begins to thicken.
5. Beat with electric mixer or rotary beater until very thick and light.

Makes about 2 cups.
Calories per tablespoon: less than 10.

Appendix

The 20 Best Sources of Selected Essential Nutrients

THE 20 BEST SOURCES OF VITAMIN A

	IU's* from 100 grams (about 3½ ounces) uncooked
Carrots	11,000
Yams	9,000
Parsley	8,500
Turnip greens	8,500
Spinach	8,100
Chard	6,500
Watercress	5,000
Red peppers	4,400
Winter squash	4,000
Egg yolk	3,400
Cantaloupe	3,400
Endive	3,300
Persimmons	2,700
Apricots	2,700
Broccoli	2,500
Pimientos	2,300
Crabmeat	2,200
Whitefish	2,000
Romaine lettuce	1,900
Mangoes	1,800

Vitamin A can also be obtained from liver (sheep, 45,000 IU's; cow, 44,000; calf, 22,000) and from cod-liver oil (200,000).

*Vitamin A is now also measured by retinol equivalents (RE's). One RE equals 3.33 IU's, or 10 IU's of beta carotene, the most common member of the carotenes.

THE 20 BEST SOURCES OF VITAMIN C

	Milligrams per 100 grams (about 3½ ounces) uncooked
Guavas	240
Black currants	200
Parsley	170
Green peppers	110
Watercress	80
Chives	70
Strawberries	57
Persimmons	52
Spinach	51
Oranges	50
Cabbage	47
Grapefruit	38
Papaya	37
Elderberries	36
Kumquats	36
Dandelion greens	35
Lemons	35
Cantaloupe	33
Green onions	32
Limes	31

Warning: **Aspirin depletes vitamin C in the body. Never take aspirin or aspirin-containing products when you're attempting to increase vitamin-C intake. If you do take such products three times a week or more, replace your vitamin-C loss with a daily supplement of 500 milligrams. Vitamin-C products containing bioflavinoids, a close chemical relative, are preferred. The ratio of vitamin C to bioflavinoids in these products should be about ten to one.**

THE 20 BEST SOURCES OF VITAMIN B$_1$ (THIAMIN)

	Milligrams per 100 grams (about 3½ ounces) uncooked
Soybeans	1.10
Sesame seeds	.98
Brazil nuts	.96
Pecans	.86

Alfalfa	.80
Peas	.80
Millet	.80
Pork	.70
Beans	.68
Buckwheat	.60
Oats	.60
Wheat	.57
Eel	.50
Hazelnuts	.46
Rye	.43
Mature sprouts	.40
Lentils	.37
Corn	.37
Rice	.34
Walnuts	.33

THE 20 BEST SOURCES OF VITAMIN B$_2$ (RIBOFLAVIN)

	Milligrams per 100 grams (about 3½ ounces) uncooked
Liver	4.10
Alfalfa	1.80
Almonds	.92
Wheat germ	.68
Mustard greens	.64
Egg yolk	.52
Cheeses	.46
Millet	.38
Chicken	.36
Mushrooms	.33
Soybeans	.31
Veal	.31
Eggs	.28
Sunflower seeds	.28
Lamb	.27
Peas	.25
Blackstrap molasses	.25
Parsley	.25
Cottage cheese	.25
Sesame seeds	.24

THE 20 BEST SOURCES OF VITAMIN B₃ (NIACIN)

	Milligrams per 100 grams (about 3½ ounces) uncooked
Peanuts	17.0
Liver	16.0
Salmon	13.0
Chicken	12.0
Tuna	12.0
Swordfish	11.0
Turkey	11.0
Rabbit	11.0
Halibut	9.2
Veal	7.8
Pork	5.5
Sardines	5.4
Sesame seeds	5.4
Beef	5.0
Potatoes	4.8
Rice	4.7
Mushrooms	4.2
Almonds	3.5
Shrimp	3.3
Peas	2.6

THE 20 BEST SOURCES OF VITAMIN B₅ (PANTOTHENIC ACID)

	Milligrams per 100 grams (about 3½ ounces) uncooked
Rice	8.9
Sunflower seeds	5.5
Soybeans	5.2
Corn	5.0
Lentils	4.8
Egg yolk	4.2
Peas	3.6

Alfalfa	3.3
Wheat	3.2
Peanuts	2.8
Rye	2.6
Eggs	2.3
Wheat germ	2.2
Blue cheese	1.8
Lobster	1.5
Cashews	1.3
Chick-peas	1.2
Avocados	1.1
Mushrooms	1.0
Chicken	.9

THE 20 BEST SOURCES OF VITAMIN B$_6$ (PYRIDOXINE)

	Milligrams per 100 grams (about 3½ ounces) uncooked
Rice	3.60
Wheat	2.90
Soybeans	2.00
Rye	1.80
Lentils	1.70
Sunflower seeds	1.10
Hazelnuts	1.10
Alfalfa	1.00
Salmon	.98
Wheat germ	.92
Tuna	.90
Bran	.85
Walnuts	.73
Peas	.67
Liver	.67
Avocados	.60
Shrimp	.60
Beans	.57
Cashews	.40
Peanuts	.40

THE 20 BEST SOURCES OF VITAMIN B₁₂ (COBALAMIN)

	Micrograms per 100 grams (about 3½ ounces) uncooked
Liver	86
Sardines	34
Clams	20
Clam broth	10
Mackerel	10
Herring	10
Snapper	9
Flounder	6
Squid	5
Hake	5
Salmon	5
Lamb	3
Octopus	3
Swiss cheese	2
Eggs	2
Haddock	2
Muenster cheese	2
Swordfish	2
Beef	2
Blue cheese	1.5

THE 20 BEST SOURCES OF FOLIC ACID

	Micrograms per 100 grams (about 3½ ounces) uncooked
Alfalfa	800
Soybeans	690
Endives	470
Chick-peas	410
Oats	390
Lentils	340
Beans	310
Wheat germ	310
Liver	290
Split peas	230

Wheat	220
Barley	210
Rice	170
Sprouts	140
Asparagus	120
Sunflower seeds	100
Collard greens	100
Spinach	80
Hazelnuts	70

THE 20 BEST SOURCES OF BIOTIN

	Micrograms per 100 grams (about 3½ ounces) uncooked
Rye	330
Soybeans	190
Liver	120
Butter	100
Split peas	82
Sunflower seeds	70
Rice	70
Rice bran	60
Rice germ	58
Egg yolk	52
Green peas	42
Lentils	42
Walnuts	40
Chick-peas	32
Barley	31
Alfalfa	30
Tuna	30
Cashews	30
Pecans	30

THE 20 BEST SOURCES OF INOSITOL

	Milligrams per 100 grams (about 3½ ounces) uncooked
Chick-peas	760
Rice	700

Wheat germ	690
Lentils	410
Pork	410
Barley	390
Veal	340
Liver	340
Oats	320
Beef	260
Beans	240
Oranges	210
Alfalfa	210
Peanuts	180
Blackstrap molasses	170
Wheat	170
Peas	160
Grapefruit	150
Sunflower seeds	150
Strawberries	120

THE 20 BEST SOURCES OF CHOLINE

	Milligrams per 100 grams (about 3½ ounces) uncooked
Egg yolk	1700
Chick-peas	780
Lentils	710
Split peas	700
Rice	650
Liver	550
Caviar	540
Wheat germ	400
Soybeans	340
Green beans	340
Peas	270
Cabbage	250
Spinach	240
Peanuts	240
Sunflower seeds	220
Sprouts	210
Blackstrap molasses	150
Alfalfa	140
Bran	140

Asparagus   130

Soy lecithin, torula, and brewer's yeasts are other excellent sources of choline.

THE 20 BEST SOURCES OF VITAMIN E

	IU's* per 100 grams (about 3½ ounces) uncooked
Wheat germ	192
Cottonseed oil	53
Sunflower seeds	37
Wheat	36
Sesame oil	31
Walnuts	26
Corn oil	25
Hazelnuts	25
Apricot oil	25
Soybean oil	19
Peanut oil	19
Almonds	18
Olive oil	17
Cabbage	10
Almond oil	10
Brazil nuts	9
Peanuts	9
Cabbage	7.8
Cashews	6
Spinach	2.9

*As natural vitamin E (d-alpha tocopherol).

THE 20 BEST SOURCES OF CALCIUM

	Milligrams per 100 grams (about 3½ ounces) uncooked
Sesame seeds	1,200
Cheeses	700
Sardines	350
Carob	350
Caviar	280
Soybeans	230

Almonds	230
Parsley	200
Brazil nuts	190
Watercress	150
Salmon	150
Chick-peas	150
Salad greens	150
Egg yolk	130
Beans	130
Pistachios	130
Lentils	130
Sunflower seeds	120
Milk	120
Buckwheat	110

Bonemeal, seaweeds, and brewer's yeast are other excellent sources of calcium.

THE 20 BEST SOURCES OF CHROMIUM

	Micrograms per 100 grams (about 3½ ounces) uncooked
Wheat	180
Vegetables	40
Fruits	30
Honey	29
Chicken	26
Parsley	21
Butter	21
Nuts	20
Grains	20
Eggs	17
Rice	16
Meats	14
Tomatoes	14
Lamb	12
Seafood	11
Pork	10
Vegetable oils	10
Beef	9
Corn	5
Carrots	3

Thyme, black pepper, cloves, and brewer's yeast are other excellent sources of chromium.

Caution: Since only an extremely small amount of chromium is absorbed by the body, supplements are recommended, particularly as GTF (Glucose Tolerance Factor).

THE 20 BEST SOURCES OF COPPER

	Milligrams per 100 grams (about 3½ ounces) uncooked
Mushrooms	6.0
Liver	4.0
Oysters	3.5
Mussels	3.0
Wheat germ	3.0
Lobster	2.0
Honey	2.0
Hazelnuts	1.5
Brazil nuts	1.0
Walnuts	1.0
Salmon	1.0
Cashews	1.0
Oats	1.0
Lentils	.5
Barley	.5
Almonds	.5
Bananas	.5
Tuna	.5
Rice	.5
Eggplant	.5

Thyme, cloves, and black pepper are other excellent sources of copper.

THE 20 BEST SOURCES OF IRON

	Milligrams per 100 grams (about 3½ ounces) uncooked
Kidneys	13.0
Caviar	12.0

Pumpkin seeds	11.0
Sesame seeds	10.0
Wheat germ	9.5
Liver	9.0
Pistachios	7.0
Egg yolk	7.0
Sprouts, mature	7.0
Sunflower seeds	7.0
Chick-peas	7.0
Millet	7.0
Lentils	6.5
Walnuts	6.0
Mussels	6.0
Oysters	5.5
Parsley	5.0
Almonds	4.5
Oats	4.5
Clams	4.0

Seaweeds, torula, brewer's yeast, and soy lecithin are other excellent sources of iron.

THE 20 BEST SOURCES OF MAGNESIUM

	Milligrams per 100 grams (about 3½ ounces) uncooked
Sunflower seeds	350
Wheat germ	320
Almonds	270
Snails	250
Soybeans	240
Brazil nuts	220
Pistachios	160
Hazelnuts	150
Pecans	140
Oats	140
Walnuts	130
Rice	120
Mushrooms	70
Chard	65
Spinach	60
Barley	55

Salmon	40
Corn	40
Bananas	30
Tuna	30

THE 20 BEST SOURCES OF PHOSPHORUS

	Milligrams per 100 grams (about 3½ ounces) uncooked
Pumpkin seeds	1,100
Wheat germ	1,100
Sunflower seeds	840
Brazil nuts	690
Sardines	580
Egg yolk	570
Walnuts	570
Soybeans	550
Almonds	500
Liver	480
Oats	410
Peanuts	400
Beans	400
Peas	400
Salmon	400
Rye	380
Lentils	380
Wheat	380
Scallops	360
Tuna	350

Soy lecithin, torula, brewer's yeast, and dolomite are other excellent sources of phosphorus.

THE 20 BEST SOURCES OF SELENIUM

	Micrograms per 100 grams (about 3½ ounces) uncooked
Corn	400
Cabbage	250

Mushrooms	140
Wheat	130
Beans	120
Peas	120
Vegetable oils	100
Onions	80
Chicken	70
Beets	65
Barley	62
Tomatoes	60
Shellfish	60
Soybeans	54
Fish, saltwater	53
Fish, fresh-water	50
Liver	50
Rice	39
Peanuts	38
Meats	22

THE 20 BEST SOURCES OF ZINC

	Zinc in milligrams per 100 grams of food, uncooked
Oysters	160
Herring	110
Wheat germ	14
Sesame seeds	10
Liver	7
Soybeans	7
Sunflower seeds	7
Egg yolk	6
Lamb	5
Chicken	5
Oats	4
Pork	3
Rye	3
Wheat	3
Corn	3
Beef	3
Beets	3
Turkey	3

Walnuts	3
Barley	3

THE 20 BEST SOURCES OF LINOLEIC ACID

	Milligrams per 100 grams (about 3½ ounces) uncooked
Safflower oil	77,000
Sunflower oil	60,000
Corn oil	54,000
Soy oil	52,000
Walnut oil	48,000
Wheat-germ oil	44,000
Sesame oil	42,000
Cottonseed oil	35,000
Sunflower seeds	30,000
Walnuts	29,000
Peanut oil	25,000
Brazil nuts	23,000
Margarine	22,000
Sesame seeds	20,000
Pecans	14,000
Peanuts	12,000
Almonds	11,000
Olive oil	10,000
Hazelnuts	9,300
Linseed oil	8,000

THE 20 BEST SOURCES OF LINOLENIC ACID

	Milligrams per 100 grams (about 3½ ounces) uncooked
Sesame oil	67,000
Linseed oil	52,000
Sesame seeds	32,000
Soybean oil	7,200
Spices	7,100

Walnut oil	6,000
Cottonseed oil	4,100
Walnuts	3,600
Soybeans	1,300
Safflower oil	1,000
Trout	1,000
Egg yolk	930
Pecans	920
Beans	750
Smelt	370
Herring	310
Sablefish	200
Lamb	190
Sole	160

THE 15 BEST SOURCES OF ARACHIDONIC ACID

	Milligrams per 100 grams (about 3½ ounces) uncooked
Walnut oil	1,600
Walnuts	960
Whitefish	480
Mackerel	470
Sole	320
Herring	310
Sardines	280
Swordfish	180
Lamb	95
Tuna	94
Mussels	90
Scallops	81
Beef	38
Cod	10
Haddock	2

THE 20 BEST SOURCES OF LYSINE

Excess lysine over arginine in milligrams, uncooked

Fresh fish, 4 ounces (salmon)	930
Shark, 4 ounces	880
Canned fish, 4 ounces	810
Chicken, 4 ounces	740
Beef, 4 ounces	720
Milk, goat's, 1 cup	520
Milk, cow's, whole, 1 cup	420
Lamb, 4 ounces	420
Mung beans, cooked, ½ cup	410
Pork, 4 ounces	380
Cheese, 1 ounce	280
Beans, cooked, ½ cup	270
Lima beans, ½ cup	240
Cottage cheese, dry curd, ½ cup	220
Mung bean sprouts, ½ cup	210
Brewer's yeast, 1 tablespoon	190
Shrimp, 4 ounces	190
Scallops, 4 ounces	190
Soybeans, cooked, ½ cup	130
Egg, 1	120

Note: **Two newly developed grains containing lysine—high-lysine corn and amaranth, a cereal that has been cultivated in South America for centuries—are both available in health-food stores.**

Glossary

All technical terms are defined where first mentioned in the text (see index). This glossary is meant to be used as a rapid refresher.

Ainsworth continuum. A graphic presentation of the degrees of sickness and health that can reveal the presence of a symptomless disease.

Antimetabolites. Drugs that treat cancer and psoriasis by interfering with the metabolic processes of the cells.

Basal-cell carcinoma. A curable form of skin cancer that affects the basal cells of the lower epidermis.

Carcinoma. A cancer that starts in the skin or mucous membranes.

Chemotherapy. A method of treating cancer by the use of poisonous chemicals.

Coal-tar derivatives. Compounds made from coal tar, used to treat some skin diseases. They may be carcinogenic.

Collagen. A protein that holds the skin together and provides its flexibility and resilience.

Corticosteroids. Drugs resembling the natural hormones secreted by the adrenal glands in the cortex. They include cortisone, and are notorious for their adverse side effects.

Dermis. The middle layer of the skin, containing essential glands, nerves and nerve endings, and blood and lymph vessels.

DNA. A double-helix structure in each cell, holding the "blueprint" for your physical and mental makeup.

EFA's. Essential fatty acids, without which the body cannot function. They are: linoleic, linolenic, and arichidonic acids.

Epidermis. The top layer of skin cells; the skin you see.

Food groups. Foods arranged in groups by the U.S. Department of Agriculture in such a way that you can plan maximum nutrient menus by making the right selections from each group.

Gamma-linolenic acid. A vital fatty acid manufactured by the body, which may be necessary as a supplement in the treatment of eczema and other diseases.

Gene. That part of the DNA that determines a specific characteristic of the body.

Hypodermis. A fatty lower layer of the skin that acts as a cushion for the rest of the skin.

Keratin. The principal component of nails, horn, hair, quills of feathers and dead skin cells.

Melanoma. A pigmented mole. A malignant melanoma is a deadly form of skin cancer.

Metastasis. The appearance of cancer in parts of the body not connected to the original tumor.

Oncogenes. Cancer-producing genes.

Oxidants. Destructive chemicals in the body that may be carcinogenic or produce carcinogens.

PGE$_1$. A hormone whose functions include the management of skin-cell production.

Polyunsaturated fats. A group of fats containing the essential fatty acids. In excess, they may form dangerous chemicals in the body unless a protective vitamin team is present.

PUVA. A conventional medical treamtment for psoriasis that combines a drug, psoralen, with ultraviolet-A radiation.

RDA. Recommended Daily Allowances of nutrients to provide maximum health.

Retinoids. Substances that are converted in the body to vitamin A.

RNA. A close chemical relative of DNA, it carries the instructions of DNA to the ribosome, the protein-producing factory in the cell.

Saturated fats. A class of fats whose main function is to supply energy. Condemned as an empty-calorie, dangerous food that, consumed in excess, can lead to degenerative diseases.

Sebaceous glands. Sometimes called oil glands, they secrete an oily substance called sebum through skin pores.

Sebum. An oily substance secreted by the sebaceous glands in the skin.

Skin system. The team of nutrients responsible for the structure and operation of the skin.

SPF. Sun Protection Factor, a number indicating how much longer you will take to sunburn with a sun-screen preparation than without protection.

Squamous-cell carcinoma. A scaly form of skin cancer that can be curable if treated in its earliest stages.

Stratum corneum. The uppermost layer of the epidermis; the "graveyard" of skin cells.

Symptomless diseases. Illness that exhibit no clinical symptoms but do reveal nutrient deficiencies.

Topical drugs. Drugs applied directly to the skin.

Triglycerides. The form fats take after being metabolized in the body.

Vitamins. Biochemicals necessary in small quantities for all bodily processes.

Recommended Reading

The following books have been selected to give the lay reader an expanded knowledge of both the conventional medical and the nutritional approaches to skin care—and of health issues in general. The works, written by specialists in their fields, are listed here under headings that, when read consecutively, form a historical summary of the nutritional-therapy revolution:

1. *The Conventional Medical Approach*
2. *The Drugs*
3. *The Nutritional Approach*
4. *The Nutrients*
5. *Cooking for Better Health*

The books have also been selected for their accessibility. Ask for them at your public library or local bookstore. (An address is provided for obtaining U.S. Department of Agriculture publications by mail.) The books we recommend have been among the sources of this work. For specific references, write to us care of Walker & Company, 720 Fifth Avenue, New York, N.Y. 10019.

The Conventional Medical Approach

Caring for Your Skin, by Jerome M. Aronberg. New York: Delair, 1981.

The Complete Medical Guide, by Benjamin F. Miller with Lawrence Galton. New York: Simon & Schuster, 1978.

Dr. Fulton's Step-by-Step Program for Clearing Acne, by James E. Fulton, Jr., and Elizabeth Black. New York: Harper & Row, 1983.

Dr. Zizmor's Skin Book, by Jonathan Zizmor. New York: Holt, Rinehart & Winston, 1977.

How to Clear Up Your Skin in Thirty Days, by Jonathan Zizmor. New York: Bantam, 1983.

Mario Badescu's Skin Care Program for Men, by Mario Badescu. New York: Everett House, 1980.

Symptoms: The Complete Home Medical Encyclopedia, edited by S. S. Miller. New York: Crowell, 1976.

Younger Skin, by Jonathan Zizmor and Sharon Sabin. New York: Holt, Rinehart & Winston, 1983.

Your Skin and How to Live in It, by Jerome Z. Litt. New York: Corinthian Press, 1980.

Your Skin, Its Problems and Care, by S. A. Zacarian. Philadelphia: Chilton, 1978.

The Drugs

AMA Drug Evaluations, edited by the AMA Department of Drugs. Chicago: American Medical Association, 1980.

The Essential Guide to Prescription Drugs, by James W. Long. New York: Harper & Row, 1980.

Non-Prescription Drugs and Their Side-Effects, by Robert J. Benowicz. New York: Berkley Books, 1982.

Physicians' Desk Reference. Oradell, N.J.: Medical Economics Company, 1984.

The Physicians' Drug Manual, edited by R. Bressler, M. Bogdonoff and G. J. Subak-Sharpe. New York: Doubleday, 1981.

United States Pharmacopeia Dispensing Information. Rockville, Maryland: The United States Pharmacopeial Convention, Inc., 1983.

The Women's Pharmacy, by Michele Paul. New York: Cornerstone/ Simon & Schuster, 1983.

The Nutritional Approach

Acne, by Kurt W. Donsback. New York: The International Institute of Natural Health Sciences, Inc., 1981.

The Book of Vitamin Therapy, by Harold Rosenberg and A. N. Feldzaman. New York: Berkley Books, 1975.

Cancer and Vitamin C, by Ewan Cameron and Linus Pauling. Palo Alto, California: The Linus Pauling Institute of Science and Medicine, 1979.

Clear Skin, by Kenneth Flandermeyer. Boston: Little, Brown, 1979.

Diet for Life, by Francine Prince. New York: Cornerstone/Simon & Schuster, 1980.

Diet, Nutrition and Cancer, edited by the National Academy of Sciences. Washington, D.C.: National Academy of Sciences Press, 1982.

Dr. Atkins' Nutrition Breakthrough, by Robert C. Atkins. New York: Bantam, 1981.

Drug Induced Nutritional Deficiencies, by Daphne Roe. Westport, Conn.: AVI Publishing, 1976.

Francine Prince's Vitamin Diet, by Francine Prince. New York: Cornerstone/Simon & Schuster, 1981.

The Healing Factor: Vitamin C Against Disease, by Irwin Stone. City TK: Grosset and Dunlap, 1972.

Health Facts, by Maryann Napoli. Woodstock, N.Y.: Overlook Press, 1981.

Healthy Living in an Unhealthy World, by Edward J. Calabrese and Michael W. Dorsey. New York: Simon & Schuster, 1984.

Jane Brody's Nutrition Book, by Jane E. Brody. New York: Norton, 1981.

Life Extension: A Practical Scientific Approach, by Durk Pearson and Sandy Shaw. New York: Warner Books, 1982.

Live or Die, by Thomas H. Ainsworth. New York: Macmillan, 1983.

Maximum Life Span, by Roy L. Walford. New York: Norton, 1983.

Medical Overkill, by Ralph C. Greene. Philadelphia: Stickley, 1983.

Nucleic Acid and Antioxidant Therapy of Aging and Degeneration, by Benjamin S. Frank. New York: Rainstone, 1977.

Nutrition, by Cheryl Corbin. New York: Holt, Rinehart & Winston, 1981.

Nutrition Against Aging, by Michael A. Weiner and Kathleen Goss. New York: Bantam, 1983.

Nutrition Against Disease, by Roger J. Williams. New York: Bantam, 1981.

Nutrition and Cancer, by G. R. Newell and N. M. Blison. New York: Raven Press, 1981.

Nutrition Guide to the Prevention and Cure of Common Ailments and Diseases, by Carlton Fredericks. New York: Fireside/Simon & Schuster, 1982.

Nutrition in the 1980's, edited by N. Selvey and P. L. White. New York: Alan R. Liss, 1981.

A Physician's Handbook on Orthomolecular Medicine, edited by R. J. Williams and D. K. Kalita. New York: Pergamon, 1977.

Supernutrition, by Richard A. Passwater. New York: Dial, 1975.

This Nutrition Business, by John Yodkin. New York: St. Martin's Press, 1976.

The Conquest of Cancer, by Virginia Livingston-Wheeler with Edmond G. Addeo, New York: Franklin Watts, 1984.

Vitamins and You, by Robert J. Benowicz. New York: Berkley Books, 1981.

The Vitamin Book, by Rick Wentzler. New York: Dolphin/Doubleday, 1979.

Your Personal Vitamin Profile, by Michael Colgan. New York: Quill/Morrow, 1982.

The Nutrients

Agriculture Handbook No. 8-1.

Agriculture Handbook No. 456.

Fats in Food and Diet.

House and Garden Bulletin No. 233.

> The above books, which contain detailed descriptions of the nutritive values of American foods, were produced by the Agriculture Research Service of the U.S. Department of Agriculture, and can be ordered by mail from the Superintendent of Documents, U.S. Government Printing Office, Washington, D.C. 20402.

Cooking for Better Health

The Dieter's Gourmet Cookbook: Low-fat, Low-Cholesterol Cooking and Baking Recipes Without Sugar or Salt, by Francine Prince. New York: Cornerstone/Simon & Schuster, 1979.

Keep It Simple, by Marian Burros. New York: Morrow, 1981.

No Salt, No Sugar, No Fat Cookbook, by Jacqueline B. Williams and Goldie Silverman. Concord, California: Nitty Gritty Productions, 1981.

Quick and Easy Gourmet Diet Recipes: Low Fat, Low Cholesterol, No Sugar, No Salt, by Francine Prince. New York: Cornerstone/Simon & Schuster, 1983.

Index

42; books about, 165–66; eczema, 55–57; herpes, 65–67; premature skin aging, 73–74; psoriasis, 48–51; skin cancer, 82–84
Cooking for better health, 108–44; books about, 168
Copper, 98, 155
Corn, 44, 71
Cortex, 49
Corticosteroids, 39, 41, 49, 50, 56, 162
Cosmetics, 105, 106
Cross-linkages, 78, 94, 98, 107
Curbing: acne, 43–46; eczema, 58–62; herpes, 68–71; premature skin aging, 76–79; psoriasis, 53–54
Cure rate(s): cancer, 84, 89, 103
Cysteine, 76, 77, 78, 87, 88, 98
Cystine, 78
Cysts, 35
Cytoxics, 85

Degenerative diseases, 25, 26, 75, 77, 81
Democycline, 104
Dermatitis, 40, 50, 63
Dermis, 3, 4, 162
Diet, 3, 4, 5, 9, 14, 39, 41, 59–60; anti-cancer, 82; average American, 8, 69, 78; nutrient-rich, 62, 77, 91. *See also* RDA diet; Supplementation (diet)
Diethylstilbesterol (DES), 86
Disease(s): symptomless, 7–8, 164
Diuretics, 104
DNA, 64, 76, 77, 81, 84, 87, 94, 107, 162, 163; and aging, 74–75
Doctors, 91, 93; supervision by, 16, 43, 44, 45, 53, 54, 58, 61, 62, 66, 68, 76, 77, 78, 88, 95–96, 99, 100, 107
Donsbach, Kurt W., 35
Drugs, 8, 41–42, 49, 66, 103–4; books about, 166; carcinogenic, 86. *See also* Side effects; Therapeutic drugs; Topical drugs
Dryness (skin), 39, 40, 43, 50, 73, 96, 103; in eczema, 55, 56, 57, 58
DTC Dome (dacarbazine), 84

Eating plan (skin), 10, 14–23
Eczema (atopic dermatitis), 55–62, 92, 95
Efudix (fluorouracil), 84, 85
Eggs, 10, 11, 27, 46, 54, 60, 78, 127
Energy, 10
Epiabrading tools, 38, 39
Epidermabrasion, 38
Epidermis, 1, 2, 4, 9, 38, 47, 73, 162
Erythromycin, 39, 104
Essential amino acids, 6, 15, 67–68, 69
Essential fatty acids (EFA's), 6, 15, 48, 52, 53, 57, 58, 61–62, 162

Estrogen, 43, 100
Etretinate, 52
Exfoliants, 38

Fat: and skin, 4
Fatigue, 8, 41, 43, 51
Fats, 6, 14, 15, 52, 107; animal, 52, 61; polyunsaturated, 25, 29, 163; saturated, 8, 25, 164
Fatty acids, 52–53. *See also* Essential fatty acids (EFA's)
Favre-Racouchot syndrome, 37, 42
Federal Dietary Guidelines for Americans, 25, 82
Fiber, 25
Fish, seafood, 11, 13, 27, 45; recipes, 112–16
Flandermeyer, Kenneth, 45
Folic acid, 59, 60, 101, 150–51
Follicles, 3, 35–36, 37, 38, 42, 50
Food additives, 60, 76
Food and Drug Administration, 38, 42, 104, 163; drug approval, 51, 66, 74; effectiveness standards, 40–42, 50, 56
Food groups, 13, 24–31, 163
Foods: best/worst for skin, 10–13, 14, 16, 24; high-cysteine, 78; nucleic-acid rich, 77; nutrient-deficient, 8, 9, 14, 26
Frank, Benjamin, 77, 78
Free radicals, 94
Fruit/Vegetable Food Group, 24, 26, 43
Fruits, 11, 13, 26, 54
Fulton, James E., Jr., 44

Gamma-linolenic acid, 57, 58, 61, 163
Garlic, 25, 46, 54
Gene(s), 81, 163
Genital regions, 40, 63
Glycerine, 105
Goldfarb, Mitchell, 82
Griffith, Richard, 68, 69
GTF (Glucose Tolerance Factor), 155

Hair loss, 41, 43, 51, 84–85
Headache, 41, 43, 51, 99
Heart attack, 25, 26, 40, 52, 99
Heavy metals, 97
Herbs/Spices Food Group, 16, 25, 30–31
Herpes, 63–71, 92, 103
Herpes simplex, 41; I, 63, 65, 67, 68, 69, 106; II, 63–64, 67, 68, 69, 106
Histamines, 56–57
Histo-compatibility complex, 74, 75, 76
Hives (urticaria), 40, 94
Hormones, 42, 43, 52; stress, 94, 100
Humectants, 105
Hyaluronidase, 89